T·A·K·E C·O·N·T·R·O·L S·E·R·I·E·S

OPERATION!
a handbook for surgical patients
Dr Robin A. J. Youngson

Books supplying expert information and practical guidance to help YOU take control

Titles published so far include

ALCOHOLISM
an insight into the addictive mind
Dr Clive Graymore

FERTILITY
a comprehensive guide to natural family planning
Dr Elizabeth Clubb and Jane Knight

SCHIZOPHRENIA
a fresh approach
Gwen Howe

DRUG ABUSE
the truth about today's drug scene
Tony Blaze-Gosden

HEALTH DEFENCE
Dr Caroline Shreeve

STROKE!
a self-help manual for relatives and carers
Dr R M Youngson

OPERATION!

A Handbook for Surgical Patients

OPERATION!

A Handbook for Surgical Patients

Dr Robin A. J. Youngson

A **David & Charles** health book

To Meredith, who makes all things possible

British Library Cataloguing in Publication Data
Youngson, Robin A. J.
  Operation!
  1. Medicine. Surgery. Operations
  I. Title II. Series
  617.91

  ISBN 0-7153-9884-9

Copyright © Dr. Robin A. J. Youngson, 1991

The right of Dr Youngson to be identified as author of this work has been asserted by him in accordance with the Copyright, Designs and Patents Act 1988.

All rights reserved. No part of this publication may be reproduced, stored in a retrieval system, or transmitted, in any form or by any means, electronic, mechanical, photocopying, recording or otherwise, without the prior permission of David & Charles plc

Printed in Great Britain
by Billings and Son Worcester
for David & Charles plc
Brunel House Newton Abbot Devon

Contents

	Preface	7
1	Diagnosis and decision	9
2	Self-preparation	25
3	Admission to hospital	36
4	The hospital staff	51
5	Tests	66
6	The anaesthetic	78
7	Consent to operation	93
8	The day of operation	104
9	Post-operative recovery	118
10	Discharge and convalescence	136
11	How to complain and sources of help	146
12	Glossary	154
	Index	159

Preface

Almost a million patients were on the UK waiting lists for surgery in 1990. Many people on the list will indeed wait for a long time and do so with mounting apprehension, in ignorance of what their operation involves. Yet little is written on the experience of going into hospital for an operation, or how you can prepare yourself for this major event.

The need for this book became apparent to me while working as a junior doctor on a surgical ward. I found many patients were bewildered and afraid, their imagination filled with the negative associations of hospital, disease, pain and suffering. The loss of personal identity in the alien hospital environment created a feeling of helplessness, excluding patients from any active participation in their treatment or recovery. But I found that simple explanations of what would happen, and why, relieved much anxiety and allowed patients to have a positive attitude. As the months went by, I spent more and more time simply explaining things.

I began to realise that as a junior hospital doctor I was in a unique position to describe what really happens on the surgical ward. The long hours spent night and day on the wards gave me an intimate view of patients' experiences, both good and bad. I learnt in considerable detail how our hospitals function and this allowed me to understand and explain some of the more bizarre and frustrating aspects of being a surgical patient. I was able to observe closely the relationship between doctors and patients and how, in some instances, patients were being denied their rights. These many experiences compelled me to write this book.

This book is for patients on a surgical waiting list. It describes in great detail what happens when you go into hospital for an operation. To make that experience more vivid, I will introduce you to four fictitious characters and through their eyes you will experience the process of diagnosis, admission to hospital, the anaesthetic, and recovery from an operation. With this knowledge, you can approach your operation with a confident and positive attitude. Throughout the book I have used clear and simple language and no prior medical knowledge is assumed.

But this book has a second aim, beyond mere description. There is a great deal you can do to prepare yourself for surgery, both mentally and physically. A successful operation depends on your active involvement at every stage, from diagnosis to post-operative recovery. Drawing on the examples of the four characters, I will explain how you can make your own decisions about surgery and how to reduce the risks of your operation. Your rights as a patient in the NHS are defined. I give a great deal of simple advice and on subjects like stopping cigarettes or losing weight, I have avoided dogmatic pronouncement in favour of explaining just how these affect your operation and anaesthetic. You must make up your own mind.

There are few benefits of a long waiting list but one is the time you now have to prepare for your coming operation. Start by reading this book.

Dr Robin A. J. Youngson

1 Diagnosis and Decision

You are on a waiting list for an operation. Quite how you got there was a simple process, at least on first inspection. You complained to your GP (general practitioner) about one or more symptoms. He decided, perhaps without going into many details, that your complaint was 'surgical' rather than 'medical' and referred you to a surgical specialist at your local hospital.

The specialist made a diagnosis and recommended an operation. You are now on the waiting list and in due course, you will have your operation and the symptoms will be cured. Simple.

In many cases, the process is just this simple and diagnosis merely involves correctly identifying a lump such as a hernia. In more complex cases, a correct surgical diagnosis is made and treated but without relieving the patient of their original symptoms. This is especially true when symptoms are of a more general nature such as abdominal pain or bowel disturbance. All medical training emphasises an approach to diagnosis in which the symptoms are fitted into a SINGLE diagnosis. The possibility of more than one diagnosis is not always contemplated and this may leave patients dissatisfied.

A study of 112 patients who underwent cholecystectomy (removal of the gall bladder, the treatment for gallstones) was presented to the British Society of Gastro-enterology in 1984. When the patients were interviewed one year after their operation, 43% rated the operation as less than successful because they still had abdominal symptoms. These included flatulence, indigestion, abdominal distension and nausea. The disappointing results of surgery are probably explained by the coexistence of two very common conditions, gallstones and irritable bowel syndrome. Gallstones may cause no symptoms whereas irritable bowel syndrome causes dyspepsia which may be mistaken for the symptoms for gallstones. When the patient is investigated, gallstones are demonstrated on a scan and assumed to be the cause of the symptoms. Because a diagnosis has been made, the surgeon need look no further because he has found something to treat. The diagnosis is the crux of western medicine without which the doctor can do little. Once a diagnosis is made, the patient can be conveniently categorised and labelled. Surgeons will often be heard referring to 'the hernia on ward seven' or 'the breast lump on ward three'. Having made a diagnosis, the treatment for that diagnosis can be prescribed. Note that the diagnosis is being treated, rather than the whole patient, and the two are not always the same thing.

In the case of the patient with two coexisting diagnoses, an operation is performed which does nothing for the irritable bowel syndrome, and symptoms recur after the operation. The operation itself may produce side effects and in the study quoted above, 27% of the patients still complained of pain in or under the scar, one year after the operation. But the process the patient went through might have been rather different. If instead of sending the patient to a surgical specialist, the GP had referred him or her to a medical specialist, a different diagnosis might have been made. Perhaps irritable bowel syndrome might have been diagnosed first, and treated with tablets or a change in diet.

The point of this discussion is to make two points. Firstly, diagnosis isn't always straightforward and a simple equation between diagnosis, treatment and patient satisfaction may not exist. Secondly, there may be a price to pay for the operation in terms of risks or side effects. In this first chapter I will explain the process of diagnosis and illustrate this with examples. I will then show you how to debate the pros and cons of your operation and tell you what questions you should ask your doctor before making up your own mind.

DIAGNOSIS

It is worth considering the process of diagnosis in more detail. This is recorded and analysed in four stages, according to a formal method taught to all doctors.

1. Presenting complaint. The doctor will record what symptoms worried you sufficiently to make you see a doctor in the first place.

2. History. The doctor will then question you closely about the onset and development of these symptoms and will also enquire after any other symptoms that you may not have mentioned or worried about. By this stage, the doctor will be on the track of one or more alternative diagnoses and will test these in the next two stages.

3. Physical examination. This elicits physical signs of disease such as swelling, tenderness and a variety of altered appearances. For instance, gall bladder disease may be suggested by the signs of yellow jaundice in the eyes and tenderness in the upper right side of the belly. Physical examination may also quantify the extent or severity of the condition.

4. Investigations. Finally, the diagnosis is confirmed by investigations such as blood tests or x-rays, although these are not always necessary.

Less experienced doctors will carry out these four steps in a formalised manner, recording all the facts in great detail. This process will be done by the ward doctor on your admission to hospital, even though the specialist has already made a diagnosis in the outpatient clinic. In the clinic, the much more experienced consultant or other surgeon will take short cuts to diagnosis. A suspected diagnosis will be confirmed by pertinent questions and limited examination and investigation. Surgical outpatient clinics are very busy places and the specialist will not be able to devote much time to your individual case. Where a diagnosis has already been made and confirmed by the GP, for instance by a scan showing gallstones, then even less time is likely to be spent with the patient.

I do not wish to belittle the very great skill and experience of consultant surgeons in this country. Such is the structure of specialist training that it may take ten or fifteen years after qualification to reach the level of consultant. Most of the surgeons I know are superb diagnosticians but there is a tendency for patients to be bulldozed into a place on the waiting list without always considering all the factors involved.

Now that I have introduced some ideas about diagnosis and the outcome of an operation, I would like to introduce you to four fictional characters whom we will follow right through the book from first symptoms to specialist consultation, and from operation to recovery. I have dramatised many of their experiences and will draw on their examples to illustrate various principles. This, of course, makes much more interesting reading and may well reflect your own experience. They all suffer from common conditions and many of you will be having the same operation as one of our characters.

Your general experience will closely resemble the examples I give but you must realise that each surgeon has individual practices which may differ from what I describe. You cannot criticise your own treatment by reference to this book.

Let's now meet the four ordinary people whose names have been drawn together for the operation list of Mr Brown, consultant surgeon, on 11 May at the Eastern Infirmary.

George Saunders. Cancer of the bowel

George is sixty-eight and is a retired engineer. He's never been busier. His wife, Mary, often says that he tries to do too much but since they moved into their new bungalow, George has really enjoyed himself. Being a highly organised and logical sort of man, he has planned a timetable for all the tasks ahead: landscaping the garden and decorating the house room by room. He keeps himself fit and well, plays golf and has been elected to the bowls team.

In the last few months he's been feeling weary and after five or six holes on the golf course he runs out of energy. On the sixth tee, at the top of a hill, he's out of breath. Mary thinks he's working too hard and keeps telling him to slow down. George is determined to stick to his timetable but feels more and more lethargic and one day Mary finds him sitting in a heap between the shafts of the wheelbarrow, looking pale and exhausted.

'Mary, I just can't do it any more!' he gasps between breaths as his pulse races.

The next few days he mopes around doing nothing and feeling depressed and irritable. Mary has noticed that he's going to the bathroom at odd times of the day.

'George, what's the matter? You always used to be regular as clockwork, right after breakfast!'

'And that's another thing,' grumbles George, 'if it's not constipation, it's diarrhoea! I don't know what's the matter with me.'

The next day he went to see Dr Barnaby and told him.

'Right! Let's have a look at you. Loosen your trousers and lie down on the couch. I want to feel your tummy.'

'Look up please,' as he gently pulled down the lower eyelid and inspected the pink lining. 'Hmm. . . I think you might be anaemic. That would explain why you're feeling so tired and short of puff. Now, just try and relax your tummy.'

Dr Barnaby felt gently but firmly around the abdomen.

'Not tender anywhere?'

'No,' said George.

Without any expression on his face, Dr Barnaby returned several times to the left side of the abdomen, feeling low down. George suddenly broke into a cold sweat as he realised that Dr Barnaby had found something on the left side. Perhaps there was a tumour gnawing its way through his insides. Was he going to die in terrible pain from cancer?

'I want to do some blood tests today, Mr Saunders, and arrange a barium X-ray of your bowel at the hospital. When you've been for the barium enema, come and see me again about three days later. I'll have a report by then and the results of the blood tests.'

'But doctor,' said George, 'is it anything serious?'

'Well,' after a pause, 'there are several possibilities but you may need an operation. Let's discuss it when I have the results. You should hear from the hospital in the next few days about the X-ray.'

Scribbling a prescription, he said, 'Take these tablets twice a day. They're iron tablets and should help to correct the anaemia. Don't worry if your bowel motions go black – that's the iron.'

George walked home in a daze. When Mary asked, he couldn't really remember what the doctor had said – something about an X-ray at the hospital.

Two weeks later he was in the outpatient clinic of Mr Brown, consultant surgeon at the Eastern Infirmary. A nurse took him into the cubicle and told him to take off his clothes, put on the dressing gown and wait. Ten minutes later, Mr Brown came in another door with a hospital file in his hands.

'Mr Saunders, how do you do? I've had a letter from your GP, Dr Barnaby. I think you've seen him since he had the results?'

'Yes,' said George.

'I want to feel your tummy, then you can get dressed and come through to my room and I'll tell you what needs to be done.' As the cool fingers probed gently on his left hand side, George began to imagine the same hands cutting and dismembering his insides. Sweat pricked on his forehead again. 'Just try and relax your tummy. Take some deep breaths.'

'Sorry!' said George. With this, Mr Brown shifted his attention to the upper right side of the abdomen and felt carefully to determine if the liver came down below the rib-cage. No, it wasn't enlarged.

'Good! Get dressed and come on through. . .'

'There's your X-ray, Mr Saunders. See here the lining of the bowel is smooth all the way around except for this patch on the left side.' His fingers stabbed at an irregular narrowing shaped rather like a chewed apple core. 'There's a partial blockage and we need to do an operation and remove it.'

'So it's not cancer, doctor?'

'Yes, I'm afraid it is. But there's no evidence of spread. I think we've caught it early, thanks to your own doctor, and you've a good chance. I want you to come into hospital next Monday and I'll do the operation on Wednesday, that's the 11 May. Any questions?'

'No,' said George, weakly.

'Right! See you next week!'

Betty Johnson. Varicose veins

Betty is forty-eight and the wife of a dairy farmer. She radiates good health and vitality and has a rosy glow in her cheeks. She's plump and cheerful and goes about her work on the farm with a good-natured bustle.

During her first pregnancy, twenty-five years before, she first began to notice some prominent veins on the back of her left calf. Over the years these had gradually become worse and she now has thick blue ropes of veins meandering down each leg. When she is up on her feet, these become very tense and bulge like grapes above her ankles. Her calves ache badly by the end of the day and the skin around her ankles has begun to thicken and discolour. On one occasion, she barked her shin on a farm gate and burst one of the veins. It bled so much she began to feel faint and called the doctor in a panic.

'Betty,' he said, 'I think it's high time you had these fixed once and for all. I'm going to send you back to Mr Brown and ask him to do an operation.'

'Can't he just inject them again?'

'No, that wouldn't work any more, Betty. Don't you worry, Mr Brown is a fine surgeon and you'll only have to stay in the hospital a day or two.'

Two months later she saw Mr Brown in the outpatient clinic.

'Hello Mrs Johnson, nice to see you again. How's Bill? Still getting up at five in the morning to milk the cows?'

'Yes, thank-you doctor. Hard work is what keeps us young and healthy! Here, I've brought you some eggs from the farm.'

'Thank-you Mrs Johnson, you shouldn't have but I know you'll not let me refuse.'

'Well doctor, you made such a lovely job of injecting the veins last time, I thought you could do them again.'

Mr Brown looked at the notes. 'Fifteen years since we first met and I've done then twice since then. Your own doctor's right, Mrs Johnson, what you need now is an operation. Oh, you could probably find someone willing to inject them but I wouldn't be honest if I pretended it would do any good.'

'Whatever you say, doctor, but I don't know how our Bill's going to manage without me,' she said doubtfully.

'Now, let's have a look. Take off your shoes and tights and stand in the light there, next to the couch. Lift your skirt please. . . Turn around. . . OK, fine! Now I want you to lie down on the couch. Let me lift your right leg up straight,' as he elevated her foot above the level of her head.

'You can't see them now, doctor, can you?'

'That's right, all the blood has drained out of the veins. Now, I'm going to put this tourniquet around the top of the thigh while I keep the leg up. . . That's it. Now, come and stand down on the floor again.' The veins in the left leg rapidly fill again but the right hand ones remain empty. Mr Brown releases the tourniquet and blood rushes down and fills the veins in a second. 'Uh, huh! That's what I suspected. The high saphenous valve is incompetent. That'll have to be tied.' And he tests the other side with the same result.

'Come and sit down Mrs Johnson. I'm going to put you on the waiting list but it will be a while before we do you. You need an operation on both legs. First we make a small cut in each groin, find the top of the vein and disconnect it. Then we can strip it out, through another small cut behind the knee. Then we make a little cut over each bulge in the veins on your calf and tease each bit out. Don't worry, we'll put you to sleep and you won't know anything about it.'

'But how will the blood get back from my feet?' she asks with consternation.

'Oh, that's all right! There's a complete system of veins deep in the leg and we'll be careful not to damage that. You see, the leg has two systems of veins rather like one-way roads. The deep vein is the main road and runs up the leg, through the groin and into the pelvis. The shallow veins are like minor roads going parallel in the same direction. At various places up the leg, there are short connecting veins like one-way streets from the minor roads to the major road. The veins have valves that only allow the blood to flow upwards or from shallow veins to deep, so it's all a one-way system.'

'In your case, Mrs Johnson, the shallow veins have become so dilated and damaged that none of the valves work any more. The blood can flow the wrong way and it pools in the bottom of the veins, blowing them up like balloons. The constant pressure can cause inflammation and further damage is done.'

'I know all about that,' said Betty. 'Sometimes a vein comes up in a hot red lump and goes hard and it's so painful!'

'That's what we call superficial thrombophlebitis.'

'I don't mind what fancy long names you call it, doctor. You put my name down for that operation and I'll come to your hospital.'

'We'll send for you but there will be a wait I'm afraid.'

'Thank-you doctor. Good day!'

The summons came thirteen months later and was then cancelled on the day of operation. No beds were available. A repeat summons came two weeks later, for 11 May.

John Reynolds. Inguinal hernia

John is a forty-nine year old storeman. For the last four months he's been getting sick notes from his doctor because of the pain and lump in his groin. He can't do any lifting because if he strains, the bulge comes down with a nasty dragging pain. He sits at home, bored stiff, and is smoking even more cigarettes than before. Like his father, he has chronic bronchitis caused by heavy smoking over many years. Each morning on waking, he has fits of coughing to clear the excess phlegm from his inflamed air passages. In the winters it gets worse, colds go down onto his chest and the phlegm becomes green and foul smelling. The coughing-fits go on all day and he often needs antibiotics to clear up the infection.

Each time he coughs, his stomach muscles tense and the pressure inside his abdomen rises. In each groin, there is a potential weakness in the abdominal wall where the spermatic cord goes through. The abdominal wall is made up of several layers and the spermatic cord passes obliquely through each along what is called the inguinal canal.

Each time John coughs, there is a pulse of pressure like a water-hammer against the opening of the inguinal canal. Gradually it began to stretch until a wide passage was created all the way down to the scrotum. If a loop of bowel is behind the opening, it can easily slide down the passage and form the hernia. Usually it goes back quite easily but sometimes it gets stuck for a while and a kink in the bowel causes a temporary blockage. John's belly begins to swell and he gets cramping pains. If he lies down flat, relaxes his tummy and gently squeezes over the lump, it usually goes back. He's learnt one or two other tricks like holding his fist over his groin when coughing, or bending his knee up to is chest. These measures stop the lump coming down.

John had never realised before how often he tenses his stomach muscles. Now he gets the familiar dragging pain in his groin to remind him. Lifting, sitting up from lying, straining on the toilet, and laughing, sneezing or coughing all bring on the pain.

In the outpatient clinic, Mr Brown was able to demonstrate the anatomy to John.

'Lie down on the couch, Mr Reynolds. I can see you have a large hernia on the left side and I suspect the beginnings of one on the right.' He listened over the lump in the groin with his stethoscope and could hear bowel sounds. That confirmed the presence of bowel in the hernia. His neat fingers deftly and gently reduced the hernia and the lump disappeared.

'Now, just one gentle cough,' as he placed his fingers over each groin to feel the water-hammer effect, what doctors call a cough impulse. 'Stand up on the floor.' With his intimate knowledge of anatomy he was able to place the tip of his forefinger exactly over the opening of the internal opening of the inguinal canal. Now, when John coughed, the pressure of his finger completely controlled the hernia and prevented it coming down.

'Lie back on the couch again.' His experienced eye had noted several signs of chest disease. John was slightly short of breath even on this negligible exertion. His fingers were tar stained, his face plethoric, the chest barrel-shaped with high square shoulders. John unconsciously pursed his lips every time he breathed out. Mr Brown tapped over John's chest with his fingers and heard the deeply resonant percussion note that is common in emphysema and bronchitis. Listening with his stethoscope he heard the coarse crackles of excess phlegm in the bronchi, and wheezes as John exhaled. A normal chest would be silent except for the faintest whisper of air movement.

He then felt for the pulses in both wrists, in each groin, behind each knee, at the ankles and on the feet. Without consciously thinking, his mind was systematically checking off the list of signs of smoking related disease. One of the grim aspects of his work was amputating legs that had become gangrenous because of blocked arteries. All such patients were smokers except for the occasional case of severe diabetes. The pulses in John's feet were weakened, indicating some early narrowing of the arteries.

'Get dressed and come and sit down. What work do you do?'

'I'm a general storeman for a component manufacturer.'

'Does that involve heavy lifting?'

'Yes, all the time.'

'So, your doctor has kept you off work?. . . Right! You need an operation to get you back to work again. We'll get you in as soon as we can, in the next few weeks.'

'We need to think carefully about an anaesthetic. The problem is that your chest is in pretty bad shape. If you needed a major operation we would take the risk of putting you to sleep but you might easily get a chest infection and that would delay your recovery. Also, we'd have to get you in to hospital several days early and work on your chest with physiotherapy, clearing the phlegm and teaching you breathing exercises. We can't justify the risk for a minor operation so we'll do it under local anaesthetic. You'll be awake during the operation and we'll freeze the tissues around the groin with injections of anaesthetic so that you don't feel anything.'

For the first time in his life, John was having to face up to the fact that his smoking was doing serious harm. He had denied any more than a smoker's cough before and had considered himself as fit as the next man.

'Is it serious, doctor? My chest, I mean.'

'Well, Mr Reynolds, I must be frank. Yes, it is potentially serious. How much do you smoke?'

'Thirty a day, but it used to be more. I've cut down.'

'Is there anyone in the family with chest disease?'

'My father had bronchitis.'

'Is he still alive?'

'No, he died when he was sixty-one.'

'Do you know what he died of?'

'I'm not sure. He kept going into hospital with his bad chest. He couldn't breathe and used to go blue. His legs swelled up and they said his heart was weak.'

'If you completely stop smoking now, your chest won't get any worse and the cough will get much better. You'll be able to enjoy your retirement. If you carry on smoking your chest will probably get worse like your father's did. You'll get more and more short of breath. You might get lung cancer. Your arteries will become narrower and you might lose the circulation to a leg. You'll double your chances of a heart attack. I can fix the hernia but if you keep on coughing like that, it'll come back again in another five or ten years. I know it's very difficult to give up smoking and I can't force you to. But those are the facts and you have to make up your own mind, which is worth more to you, your health or the enjoyment of smoking? I'm not going to refuse to treat you just because you can't give up smoking.

I'll write to your doctor and tell him that you're on the waiting list. I think you should go and see him and talk through the smoking business.'

'Oh! He's always going on about my smoking,' said John, 'but I never really believed him. When you said my chest was too bad for an anaesthetic, it gave me a fright, it made me realise. Thank you, sir, I'll do my best for you!'

'No, Mr Reynolds, it's for you.'

'Well, er, yes, doctor. Thank you doctor.'

Susan Williams. Gallstones

Susan is an attractive thirty-four year old mother of two small children. She had always taken care of her figure, went to weekly aerobic classes and was a stylish dresser. These qualities had contributed to her success as personal assistant to the managing director of a local company. She had a particular flair for organisation.

Apart from very brief stays when she delivered the two babies, she had never been in hospital and was proud of her fitness and health. She was therefore alarmed and dismayed when the trouble began five months earlier.

The first bout occurred when the family was on holiday in Spain. They had been out for a meal and as she put the children to bed she began to feel uncomfortable in her upper abdomen. She put it down to indigestion. However, the feeling didn't go away and later when she was in bed, it began to get worse. Over about an hour it became very severe, a constant sharp pain right across the top of her tummy. Susan rolled about in bed, arms wrapped around herself, her knees drawn up and sweating profusely. She was sick once. She didn't trust a local doctor and didn't fancy being poked around by someone who couldn't even speak English. She thought it must be food poisoning and that it would pass off. But when the pain became really bad she agreed to let her husband find a doctor.

After several calls on the 'phone, he managed to find the name of a doctor used by the local branch of his company and was assured that his travel insurance would foot the bill.

The doctor came and was very polite and efficient. He wasn't sure what the cause was, an ulcer or gallstone, but gave her rapid relief with an injection of pethidine, and an anti-emetic to stop the nausea. He was quite willing to admit her to his clinic for investigation the next day but in the morning, Susan felt quite well again and decided to return to England.

Her own doctor didn't seem concerned. 'Probably just a bout of gastro-enteritis,' he said. Susan had no recurrence of the severe pain but was troubled by a lot of indigestion and after a while, realised that it usually followed a fatty meal. When she excluded fat and oil from her diet, the symptoms resolved. She felt in control again.

A month later, Susan had some mild discomfort and then began to feel unwell. She felt nauseated, lost her appetite and the whites of her eyes went slightly yellow. She went to see her doctor determined to persuade him that something was seriously wrong. She had kept notes of the symptoms in her diary.

'Hmm. Sounds like gallstones. Tell me, has there been any change in the colour of your bowel motions or urine?'

'Yes, my water went dark and bowel motions light in colour.'

'Very smelly and difficult to flush because they float?'

'Yes!' said Susan in surprised agreement.

'Right, Oh! You just slip off your skirt and lie down there and I'll fill in the form for liver function tests. That's a type of blood test.'

'Liver!' said Susan, slightly alarmed. 'I thought you said gallstones?'

'So I did, young lady. But if a gallstone blocks the bile duct, it causes back pressure on the liver which results in inflammation, and jaundice. The blood test will measure the jaundice and tell me if there is any inflammation of the liver.'

He inspected the whites of her eyes and noted the faint tinge of yellow. Palpating gently in the abdomen, he found that Susan tensed slightly whenever he felt under the ribs on the right side. 'Hmm. A bit tender there?'

In answer to a buzzer on his desk, the nurse came in.

'Ah, Jean! Can you find me a 5ml syringe, green needle and plain clotted bottle, please?. . .'

'Don't move your arm. Sharp scratch coming up. . . There!. . . Press on that for a minute then put your things on again. I'll write a letter to George Brown at the Infirmary and ask him to see you.' Picking up his fountain pen, he wrote:

Dear George,

I would be grateful if you could see this young lady whom I think has gallstones. Although she is a little young for this complaint, she gives a good history of one attack of biliary colic, followed by fatty dyspepsia. She has presented to me today with some mild obstructive jaundice that appears to be resolving. On examination, she is tender in the right hypochondrium.

She is a sensible and intelligent lass who otherwise keeps herself in good health. No significant PMH. Her only medication is the pill.

20 · Diagnosis and Decision

I know you like to document these cases before considering cholecystectomy so I have sent off some LFTs today and I will arrange an u/s scan of the liver and gall-bladder.

I look forward to your opinion.

With best wishes,

Andrew Holden.

'I understand most of that,' said Susan, 'but what's PMH?'
'Past Medical History.'
'I presume cholecystectomy is removal of the gall-bladder?'
'Yes, that's right.'
'And u/s? Is that ultrasound scan?'
'Yes, the same as you had when you were pregnant. Not just for looking at babies, you know. So wait until you hear from the hospital about the scan and George will see you soon after that. He's pretty quick off the mark when someone's having trouble with gallstones. When you've seen him, visit me again. If you get that bad pain again, or go yellow, or get a fever, get in touch with me quickly, OK? Oh, and you'd better stop the pill.'
'Why? Does it make gallstones worse?'
'Possibly, but it does increase the risk of blood clots in the legs after surgery.'
'Thrombosis, you mean?'
'Yes, that can be dangerous. What are you going to do about contraception in the meantime? You can go back on the pill afterwards.'
'I've still got the cap at home,' said Susan.
'Any other questions?'
'No, thank you, Dr Holden. I feel much happier now that something is being done. Goodbye!'
'Bye!'

The outpatient clinic

This is the only routine access to specialist opinion that GPs have for their patients. Referral is made by letter to a chosen consultant. He will read all referral letters and will assign priority to the cases according to the information supplied by the GP. There is a waiting list for outpatient appointments and while urgent cases may be seen within a week or two, others may wait several months. Appointments are made well in advance so you should be notified of your appointment soon after your GP has written. No reply is sent to the GP until the patient has been seen in the clinic, when a letter will be written detailing the diagnosis and what treatment is planned. This letter to the GP is often delayed by ten days because it is dictated, has to be typed, then checked by the doctor at the following clinic, then posted.

If a very urgent referral is needed, then your GP will telephone the hospital and speak directly to the consultant. Admission can even be arranged on the same day and this is how surgical emergencies, such as acute appendicitis, are handled, bypassing the outpatient clinic.

From the patient's point of view, outpatient clinics often seem to be inefficiently organised and many complain that they have to wait an hour or two for a very short appointment. The reason for this is simple. The clinics take up a large proportion of a surgeon's time, more than he spends in the operating theatre. Very large numbers of patients are seen and all the surgeons will work non-stop through the clinic. Each consulting room is surrounded by several examination cubicles so that while the surgeon is seeing one patient, another is undressing ready for him. The whole clinic is organised so that a continuous supply of patients is presented to the surgeon. On any day, some patients will fail to attend and some will be late for their appointment. Therefore to avoid any gaps in the supply of patients, appointments are bunched up near the beginning of the clinic.

Because the clinics are so busy, there is little time to discuss the operation. This is very unsatisfactory for the reasons I will now discuss.

DECISION

I expect that most of you reading this book are now in the position of George, Betty, John or Susan. In other words, you're on the waiting list for an operation. Not many of you will yet have a definite date for the operation and I would warn you that it may well come at short notice. Ironically, the longer you wait, the shorter the notice you may get. Although this seems daft and an example of poor organisation, there is an explanation that I will go into later.

The period of waiting can be very trying. But there are ways in which you can use this time positively, to promote rapid recovery after the operation and to minimise the disruption to your work and private life.

Firstly, you must make sure that it is YOUR decision to have the operation. That sounds an odd thing to say. 'Of course I have decided to have an operation!' But when I first started work on the surgical wards as a newly qualified doctor, I was surprised to discover that almost none of the patients had DECIDED to have an operation. They had gone to their doctor with a complaint, he'd referred them to a surgeon, the surgeon said he would do an operation and here they were! It was a case of blind faith. Very few knew what the operation involved and although some were squeamish and didn't want to know, many were curious but hadn't felt able to ask. They hoped that the surgery would put right whatever complaint they presented to their doctor but few had any precise idea of what the benefits of the operation would be. In an ideal world, all these topics would be discussed in the outpatient clinic but this rarely happens, mostly because there isn't time.

The balance of risk and benefit

It has to be realised that every operation or medical treatment carries a certain risk — as does the condition being treated. Every time a doctor writes a prescription or does an operation he has to weigh up the balance of risk and benefit. That risks are involved in surgery seems obvious because we are all aware of the highly publicised disasters in the medical world that attract huge compensation claims. In 1987, for the first time in this country, a court awarded damages in excess of a million pounds. But the equation may be more subtle, and bad decisions made much more often than we think. Cholecystectomy (removal of the gall-bladder) is an example I discussed earlier in this chapter. The benefit of this operation cannot always be taken for granted even if the risks of operating are thought to be small.

The ill effects of an operation are called complications. Some complications may be very rare, but the equation must take into account how serious the complication is if it does occur. For instance, very rarely after cholecystectomy, one of the internal stitches might come undone allowing a leak of bile into the peritoneal cavity. This can cause a life threatening condition called biliary peritonitis which might require a second, emergency operation and a period in intensive care.

Treatment with medicines can be equally hazardous, particularly in the elderly. It is shocking to realise that 20% of hospital admissions in the elderly are caused by side effects or adverse reactions to the medicines they are taking. There was a good example in my own hospital last week. An elderly lady was admitted, unable to care for herself any longer because of vomiting, diarrhoea and repeated falls. She became so giddy that she fell down the stairs and broke her hip. It didn't take long to establish that her weakness and giddiness were caused by severe anaemia (a dilution of the blood caused by a deficiency of haemoglobin, the red substance that carries oxygen). She told us that her doctor had started her on a new arthritis pill six weeks before and these had caused severe indigestion. This was a clue to the cause of her anaemia and when the lining of her stomach was directly visualised through a gastroscope, suspicions were confirmed. The tablets had inflamed the stomach and she had eventually formed an ulcer. The ulcer was slowly bleeding, causing the anaemia and diarrhoea. I'm pleased to say that she made a full recovery.

Although a bleeding stomach ulcer is a very rare complication of this sort of tablet, because arthritis is so common in the elderly, millions are taking this or similar medicine. You might think that a risk of 1 in 10,000 was acceptable for the individual but that represents thousands of adverse reactions when so many prescriptions are written.

So, having illustrated the point with some examples, we can think about the balance of risk and benefit of your operation and what you need to know to make your own decision.

THE QUESTIONS YOU NEED TO ASK

First of all, you need to know more about your condition. Is it serious? Will it get better or worse on its own? How long does it last?

Like the characters in this book, you are already aware of some of the unpleasant effects of your condition but it is unlikely that you have experienced the full range of symptoms. Some conditions which cause few symptoms may carry a risk of serious complications. Is there an alternative treatment that doesn't involve surgery?

The answers to these questions are very different for the conditions suffered by George, Betty, John and Susan. It is important to realise that the operation may only partly improve some symptoms and not influence others at all. Conversely, some conditions can be completely cured. Betty is bothered a lot by aching in her calves at the end of the day. Does she realise that the varicose vein operation may not improve this at all? George has cancer and is afraid of dying young. Is the operation going to improve his chances of survival?

You need to know a lot more about the operation and its complications. Some complications are common and predictable and of only minor importance. This includes the external scar. Will Susan still wear a bikini after her operation? Other complications are much less common, unpredictable and may be serious. This includes failure of the operation. An example is vasectomy where by some incredible chance (1 in 6000) the cut-and-tied ends of the vas manage to join together again, restoring fertility.

The very best person to answer these technical questions is the surgeon and, if he is wise, he will already have made sure you understand the important points. Otherwise, he's going to have a lot of disappointed customers. Unfortunately, the busy outpatient clinic rarely gives sufficient time to discuss these issues and unless you went very well prepared, you have probably missed that opportunity.

The next best person is your own GP and he or she is well qualified to discuss these and wider issues. All doctors are taught and examined in surgery as students, and even GPs have to work in a surgical post for a minimum of six months after qualification. Many GPs also have experience in the surgical specialities such as orthopaedics and gynaecology. GPs also play an important role in the post-operative care and convalescence of patients after discharge from hospital, and in the treatment of minor complications. Your own doctor has sent many patients for operation and will have seen the results. He is entitled to refer his patients to any surgeon of his choosing within the district and sometimes beyond. Over the years, he is likely to have built up a relationship with a small number of surgeons whom he trusts and respects.

Your own doctor is therefore in a very good position to advise you on most aspects of an operation and if he knows you well, will be able to anticipate and answer many of your fears. To make sure you don't forget any questions when you see your GP, write a list to take with you.

One factor I haven't mentioned so far is the risk of the anaesthetic. This is discussed fully in Chapter six which explains how an anaesthetic works. For the average patient, the risk of death or brain damage due to the anaesthetic alone is almost infinitely small. You are probably at greater risk during your journey to hospital! In summary, you want the answers to five questions:

- What are the other symptoms I might suffer with this condition?
- If I don't have the operation, will this condition get better or worse and might I suffer any serious complications?
- Which of the above will be cured or prevented by the operation?
- What are the possible complications of the operation and how likely are they?
- Is there an alternative treatment?

With the answers to these questions you can now make up your own mind. Don't be afraid to cancel an operation if, on reflection, the balance of risk and benefit aren't right for you. This is an area of subjective judgement which depends on the values you give to various possible outcomes. This subject is discussed more fully in chapter seven which deals with consent to operation.

If you do cancel, you should do it well in advance and with the consultation of your own doctor. The surgeon won't mind and will understand that circumstances can change during the long wait on the list. He will still have your notes and details and at the request of your own doctor, he can see you again, or put your name back on the list.

You also have the right to a second consultant opinion but this will require a new referral letter from your GP. This is not a frequent occurrence and is almost always the result of poor communication or inadequate explanation. You may get slightly different answers to your five questions but as the values that you place on the relative risks and benefits are your own, you are unlikely to come to a different conclusion.

The next chapter tells you how to prepare yourself for surgery and improve the balance of risk and benefit.

2 Self-Preparation

In the first chapter I introduced you to the idea of balancing risk against the benefit of your operation. Until now, the factors you considered in making your decision have simply been the facts of the case. The important message of this chapter is that you have the power to influence many of these factors and tip the balance much more in your favour.

You might imagine that your operation is rather like fixing a car. After all, the fault in a car has to be diagnosed, rather like your condition, and then put right by an operation which delves into the innards. But the analogy is false. The motor car is a purely passive object in which the outcome of the operation is determined the moment repair is finished. In contrast, your operation is only the beginning of a long process of interaction between the treatment, and your mind and body.

You have two goals: a successful operation and a rapid, uncomplicated recovery. Each depends on the other. Self-preparation is crucial to these goals and there is a great deal you can do to reduce the risk of surgery and promote recovery. One of the few benefits of a long waiting list is the opportunity it gives you for preparation. Start now because you may be called for your operation at any time.

I will consider the subject under a number of headings:

- Mental attitude
- Physical fitness
- Nutrition
- Obesity
- Smoking
- Alcohol
- Medications
- Dental treatment.

MENTAL ATTITUDE

Lying in bed is dangerous and is even sometimes fatal! This is especially true after an operation. Some of the reasons for this are explained later in the book but for the moment, take my word for it. It is very noticeable when looking at the behaviour of patients after an operation, that some are 'go-ers' and others are determined to display an attitude of great suffering

26 · Self-Preparation

and immobility. The 'go-ers' are sitting up in bed soon after an operation, looking alert and cheerful, demanding to know when they can eat, get out of bed and go home. They have a few doses of pain-killers and then refuse any more. In contrast, the 'loungers' lie in bed like a sack of potatoes, demand numerous doses of pain-killers and are very slow to mobilise. The worrying aspect is that the latter group suffer more complications and are less likely to make a good recovery. They spend longer in hospital. The most dramatic example of the effects of this division is in the recovery of elderly women after emergency operation for fractured hips. The elderly are at greatest risk of post- operative immobility and every effort is made to get these patients back on their feet within days. Those that walk in the first week usually make a full recovery; those that don't often linger and even die in the following weeks or months.

This is not to say that I think pain-killers are a bad thing and I certainly wouldn't like you to suffer on that score. But I'm trying to explain the fundamental difference in attitude these two groups have towards their operation and recovery. Don't underestimate the effects of your mind on healing and recovery. Every doctor has seen patients who by the strength of their will have survived or died against all predictions. I remember an elderly female patient in whom lung cancer was newly diagnosed. Although this was not advanced, it was not a suitable case for surgery. The tumour was small and she might confidently be expected to remain in good health for at least some months. However, in her own mind, cancer was an immediate death sentence and she merely waited for confirmation of the diagnosis.

'It is cancer, isn't it, doctor?'

'Yes.'

'I don't wish to live any more. I'm going to die. Can I please stay in the hospital?'

'Well, of course you can stay a few days but there's no reason why you can't go home and enjoy good health for a while.'

'Please don't send me home! Let me stay!'

On the evening six days later, she made her farewells. She refused to complete a menu card for breakfast the following morning. She died peacefully that night with no apparent reason for her early demise other than her determination to die.

On the same ward was an elderly lady with advanced cancer of the womb which had spread within her abdomen and caused a complete blockage of her bowels. She was given morphine for the pain and was expected to die within a day or two. Six months later, when I moved on to a different posting, she was established as a lively and permanent resident on the ward. She had received no treatment for the cancer other than her determination to survive.

In a later chapter which talks about your anaesthetic, I describe some experiments that show the power of the mind over pain. I'm not talking about Indian mystics or advanced practitioners of yoga but about ordinary people.

Each of us has, within ourselves, more mending and healing powers than most of all the medicines put together. Part of the success of 'alternative' medicine is that it addresses the natural healing powers within us. The responsibility for healing is put back in the patient's hands rather than saying, 'You have a disease. You are helpless to do anything about it but I can cure you with this tablet/operation.'

So, this is my prescription: You must take responsibility for yourself. Your operation is going to be a success and your recovery rapid because you are determined to take charge. I want you to imagine that you have had your operation. I want you to visualise, in the mind's eye, your body fit and strong. The pain or disfigurement or disability is gone and your body is whole again. I want you to imagine the feeling of relief and the pleasure in being well. I want you to imagine your rapid recovery and boasting to your friends, 'Well, of course, I'm a very fast healer.' I want you to imagine the doctors standing at the end of your bed after your operation and saying to each other, 'Mrs . . . (or Mr . . .) is certainly a 'go-er'. She'll do well.' And then I want you to imagine how you will go into hospital relaxed and confident, knowing what to expect after reading this book. Practise this visualisation exercise regularly.

PHYSICAL FITNESS

You'll be glad to hear that I'm not going to recommend five-mile jogs or weight-training in the gym! In fact, the super-fit have a disconcerting tendency of requiring more anaesthetic to put them asleep and of waking up very rapidly after the anaesthetic and climbing off the bed! So long as you can walk a mile on the flat or climb a couple of flights of stairs briskly without becoming very short of breath, you are fit enough for your operation.

If you cannot manage even this level of exertion, you must talk to your own doctor about your general health and fitness. He will also want to know if you get any pain or tightness in your chest when you exert yourself. He should examine your heart and chest and he may decide to arrange an ecg (electrocardiogram, a tracing of your heart's electrical rhythm recorded in a few minutes by a simple machine through wires attached to your wrists and ankles). This doesn't, of course, apply if you are unable to walk or climb stairs because of severe arthritis. If your doctor finds nothing wrong he will probably recommend that you take up some gentle exercise such as regular walks.

Perhaps you already have a chest or heart condition diagnosed and your doctor will have mentioned this to the surgeon. Sometimes, the surgeon will arrange for the patient to see one of the medical specialists at the hospital prior to the operation. Otherwise, the admitting doctor at the hospital will assess your general health with questions and a complete physical examination. In many hospitals, it is routine practice to do an ecg and chest x-ray on any patient over 55 or 60. Having said all this, the huge majority of you will be perfectly fit for an anaesthetic and operation. Even if you do have a medical condition, don't worry. Elderly and sick patients are routinely and safely given anaesthetics nowadays.

However, there is one common circumstance in which some simple exercises, even for the fit, are beneficial. If you are having an abdominal operation, the incision will cause at least a temporary weakening in the wall of the abdomen. The extent of this will depend on the site and length of the incision. The wall of the abdomen is a muscular structure and its strength depends almost entirely on the development of these muscles. In the elderly and the very unfit, these muscles may become so weak that the contents of the abdomen begin to bulge out in unsightly lumps. This is much more common in the overweight. After an abdominal operation this may become a serious problem with the formation of a hernia where some of the bowels push between the muscles and form a swelling under the skin.

This almost never happens in slim patients with reasonable tummy muscles. So, next time you have a bath, stand up and have a look at the shape of your tummy. If the tummy muscles are very soft and your belly sags a little, then you need to tone up the muscles with some simple exercises. This need not be at all strenuous.

For those with a very lazy tummy, the easiest exercise is lifting the head and shoulders off the floor when lying flat on your back. Do this a few times and it's surprising how quickly the muscles begin to shake and tremble. Regular practice for just a minute a day will soon reap dividends. For the fitter or more ambitious, this can be extended to sit-ups from the same position. For the positively masochistic, the exercise simply involves lying flat on your back holding your feet six inches off the floor!

The common cold
This is a convenient point to mention this most frequent cause of temporary ill health. A cold will increase the risk of chest infection after a general anaesthetic. If you are due to have anything more than a very minor operation, this should be postponed until you have fully recovered from the cold. If you feel at all unwell, are feverish or have a chesty cough, then ANY operation, however minor, should be postponed if a general anaesthetic is required.

What should you do in this circumstance? The letter inviting you to the hospital for an operation is usually sent only a few days beforehand. If you are obviously unwell, ring the hospital admissions office (the phone number will be on the letter) and tell them. They will cancel your admission and inform the surgeon who will probably try and get another patient to come in your place. This is why it is important to ring as soon as you can. No one will mind and your operation will be rescheduled a week or two later when you have had a chance to recover. This is much better than going through the whole process of admission to hospital only to be sent home again without an operation.

If you have a bit of a runny nose but otherwise feel perfectly well and you are having a minor operation, then don't worry. The operation can almost certainly go ahead.

If you fall somewhere in between these two examples, you will need further advice. First of all, ring the admissions office of the hospital. This is the least trouble and may give you a quick answer. Failing this, or on the advice of the hospital, you should go and see your own doctor. He may want to inspect your throat or listen to your chest and will be able to advise you.

The same advice applies to any other minor malady.

NUTRITION

Any operation places a stress on the body and a period of healing and recovery is required to regain full health and fitness. This is a complex process of tissue repair, replacement of lost body fluids and blood, and of fighting infection.

Tissue repair and wound healing require an ample supply of protein, fats and an energy source such as carbohydrate. If these are not adequately supplied by a balanced diet, then healthy tissues in the body will be broken down to provide the essential ingredients. This causes weakening and wasting of the body in general and of the muscles in particular. A poorly nourished person will be slow to heal. In a severely debilitated patient, this process can even contribute to kidney failure because the waste products of tissue breakdown overload the excretory capacity of the kidney. In addition, a number of vitamins and trace elements are essential for healing. For example, iron, vitamin B12 and folate are all essential requirements for the replacement of lost blood by the bone marrow. A deficiency of vitamin C slows healing and if severe, can actually cause bruising and bleeding. This is one of the signs of scurvy, the vitamin C deficiency disease suffered by sailors of old. Likewise, a deficiency in zinc also impairs healing. Copper is required by the white blood cells of the immune system and a shortage of copper reduces their number, making infection more likely.

Causes of a poor diet

The majority of people in this country consume an excess of protein and carbohydrate and are certainly not malnourished in that sense. However, some people's diet is deficient in minerals, particularly if they eat a lot of 'junk' food and little fresh fruit and vegetables. Alternatively, your surgical condition may have caused a loss of appetite with a poor diet for that reason. The 'tea and toast' diet of some elderly people living alone may also have serious deficiencies. If you cannot manage a balanced diet for any of these reasons then I would advise you to seek the advice of your doctor or local pharmacist and consider supplements of vitamins and minerals.

Constipation

There is another, more mundane reason for considering your diet prior to an operation and that is constipation! Even people with a regular bowel habit often find that a stay in hospital leads to constipation. There are several reasons for this including a period of immobility, disruption of your normal daily routine and sometimes the effects of the operation itself. The best prevention of constipation is a diet rich in fibre, found in fresh fruit and vegetables, cereals and wholemeal bread. Getting to the toilet in a hurry on the hospital ward after an operation may not be the easiest of tasks so laxatives are not a practical solution to the problem. Make a habit of eating more fibre and try and continue this in hospital. The bowl of fruit brought by hospital visitors is not such a bad idea after all!

OBESITY

Like smoking, obesity causes problems by degree. Patients who are a little overweight will have no problem and those who are grossly obese may be refused their operation because their surgical condition doesn't warrant the increased risk of an operation and anaesthetic. I recall a young woman of seventeen stone whose surgeon refused to perform a gall-bladder operation until she lost weight. In fact her case will serve well to illustrate the difficulties caused by obesity.

Several months after the initial consultation she was admitted to the hospital as an emergency with severe abdominal pain. One of the gallstones had become impacted in the neck of the gall-bladder causing a blockage and severe inflammation. It was decided to operate on her the next day.

As a consequence of her obesity, she developed a hiatus hernia and quite often had heartburn. When she lay flat in bed, stomach acid sometimes came all the way up to her mouth. The anaesthetist was afraid this might happen when he was putting her to sleep and so had to modify his anaesthetic technique to take account of this risk. This made the anaesthetic more complicated.

It was difficult to find a vein in her arm to site the intravenous 'drip' and he was only successful in inserting the needle at the second attempt. The moment she was asleep, he inserted a tube into the windpipe and this was awkward to perform because her neck was so fat. Because of her large body size, he had to use much bigger doses of anaesthetic drugs and he knew she would be slower to wake up than a slim patient.

It required four people to lift her from the anaesthetic trolley onto the operating table. The gall bladder was a long way down a deep hole through all the tummy fat and this made the operation difficult. The skin cut had to be bigger to compensate. In common with any obese patient, her innards were also covered in layers of fat, further increasing the difficulty of the operation which took twice as long as usual. It is very difficult to sew fat together so the skin stitches has to be made extra large to strengthen the wound. The anaesthetist liked to use an epidural infusion to relieve pain after the operation but did not attempt it in this case because he couldn't feel the backbone where the epidural injection is placed. Ordinary injections of pain-killer had to be made with extra long needles to pass through the fat on her legs.

She made a surprisingly good post-operative recovery with only a minor chest infection requiring antibiotics. One end of the wound came slightly apart but eventually healed well. Because of her great size and immobility, she was especially at risk of developing deep venous thrombosis (blood clots in the legs). To reduce this risk, she had thrice daily injections under the skin of a drug that reduces blood clotting.

In summary, she had a safe anaesthetic and operation entailing a number of extra precautions and relative difficulties. Neither the anaesthetist nor the surgeon particularly enjoyed the case though they were both skilled and experienced in the management of obese patients. Not all cases go so well.

What does scientific research show?

A study of the risks of moderate obesity during surgery was published in the British Medical Journal in July 1988 by researchers at Northwick Park Hospital. They studied almost 500 patients having abdominal operations and looked to see if those with moderate obesity suffered an excess of complications post-operatively. 73 of the 500 patients were at least 30% overweight by comparison with the ideal weight for their height. The obese patients were found to have a much higher risk of wound infections with an incidence of 43% when compared with the non-obese group with a 25% incidence. They found no difference in the rates of other complications. Remember, this study applied only to patients with moderate obesity (of the order of two or three stone overweight) and the researchers acknowledged the special problems of more severely obese patients.

If you are overweight, I would strongly advise you to try and lose weight before your operation. One of the few advantages of a long waiting list is that you have time to lose weight gradually. Don't go on a crash diet. Aim to lose weight very gradually, only a pound or two a week, and you are much more likely to succeed. Quite apart from your operation, losing weight will reduce your chances of developing diabetes, high blood pressure and arthritis of the hips, amongst many other medical conditions associated with obesity.

SMOKING

The most important thing you can do for yourself before your operation is to stop smoking.

Fact: following operations on the abdomen, smokers are SIX times as likely to suffer from post-operative chest complications as non-smokers. This was established more than 40 years ago. There is also evidence that smoking may interfere with wound healing and also alters the metabolism of drugs amongst many other effects. Fortunately, some of the harmful effects of smoking last only a few hours or days so giving up for even a short time will benefit you. Let me explain:

Cigarette smoke contains a poisonous gas called carbon monoxide. A molecule of carbon monoxide is almost the same shape and size as a molecule of oxygen. Every cell in the body needs a regular supply of oxygen to survive. Oxygen molecules are carried in the blood by large protein molecules which make up the substance called haemoglobin. This is the substance that colours blood red. Each molecule of haemoglobin is rather like a container lorry. It arrives at the lungs, picks up four molecules of oxygen, delivers them to a distant part of the body and then returns empty to the lungs to complete the round trip. We could not survive without haemoglobin in the blood and a relative deficiency of haemoglobin is called anaemia. Because the molecules of carbon monoxide are so similar to oxygen, they also latch on to haemoglobin, in place of oxygen molecules. The problem is, they get stuck there. Even if the concentration of carbon monoxide in the lungs is very low, the concentration in the blood builds up and fewer haemoglobin molecules are available to carry oxygen. So, the vital supply of oxygen to the tissues is reduced and wound healing is slowed.

Cigarette smoke also contains nicotine, a powerful drug. One of the effects of this drug is to make the heart muscle work harder and consume more oxygen. Ordinarily, this doesn't matter, but if you have been smoking a long time, you may have narrowing of the coronary arteries which supply blood, and therefore of oxygen to the heart muscle. There is usually a balance between the consumption and supply of oxygen to the heart muscle. The combined effect of carbon monoxide and nicotine in cigarette smoke may worsen this balance by as much as 25%. Anaesthesia and surgery place a strain on the heart and in severe cases, this 25% difference might tip the balance far enough to cause a heart attack (coronary). It is crucial that any patient who suffers from angina (chest pain caused by lack of oxygen supply to the heart muscle) avoids smoking for 24 hours before their operation. It takes 12-24

Self-Preparation · 33

hours to eliminate carbon monoxide and nicotine from the blood. I would strongly advise any smoker to follow the same advice.

Other effects of smoking on the chest last longer, such as predisposition to chest infection. Every one of us inhales dirt and germs into our lungs every day. One reason we don't all get pneumonia is because the airways in the lungs have a very efficient method of clearing out small particles. The lining of the airways has a microscopic surface rather like a field of wheat. In the same way that the wind creates ripples that travel across the field as wheat stalks sway, the tiny finger-like cilia that line the airways beat in synchronization to create waves that travel up towards the throat. Sticky mucus secreted by specialised cells traps the particles and this is gently wafted up to the throat and usually swallowed.

Cigarette smoke directly inhibits the beating of the cilia and reduces the clearance of germs. The germs have time to multiply and a chest infection can result. If you stop smoking for several days, the cilia can recover and a chest infection is less likely after the operation.

Regular smoking causes bronchitis. This simply means inflammation (-itis) of the air passages (bronchi). The effect of this is gross enlargement of the mucus-secreting cells which then produce abnormally large amounts of mucus. This is the cause of the increased volumes of phlegm produced by smokers and the reason for the smoker's morning cough. The continual inflammation gradually causes permanent damage to the cells lining the bronchi, and cilia are lost leaving bare patches. In consequence, the large volumes of phlegm tend to stay in the chest and this also makes infection more likely. It takes one to two weeks for the volume of mucus to reduce after smoking is stopped.

These effects may be made much worse by the anaesthetic and operation. If you have a lot of phlegm in the chest when you have an anaesthetic, this can block some of the small airways. This prevents air getting to the parts of lung beyond the blocked airways, which then collapse, often causing a focus of infection. If, in addition, you have had an abdominal or chest operation, coughing will be painful. If you don't cough and clear the phlegm, a pneumonia may result. One of the jobs of physiotherapists, whom you will meet later in the book, is to try and prevent this situation by teaching breathing exercises and assisting your coughing.

It is estimated that if you want to get the maximum benefit from stopping smoking before your operation, you must stop four to six weeks beforehand.

Having said all this, it must be admitted that most smokers who are otherwise fit come through their operation and anaesthetic perfectly well. The difference can be seen in the recovery ward immediately after the operation where many of the smokers are having coughing fits while their non-smoking fellow patients recover quietly and smoothly from the anaesthetic.

If you are having a major abdominal operation do think carefully about it. I have seen more than one patient with chronic bronchitis suffer serious complications. They developed pneumonia which reduced the amount of oxygen in the blood. This delayed healing and weakened the surgical wound. Finally, with the continual stress of coughing the wound burst open requiring a second operation to sew it up again. This is a slippery slope to find yourself on.

ALCOHOL

When you are admitted to hospital, the doctor will ask you how much alcohol you drink. This is not to be nosey or make any moral judgement but because your alcohol consumption may make a difference to your treatment. Any person who can 'hold their drink' has become tolerant to the effects of alcohol and will not notice the symptoms of drunkenness until they have consumed more alcohol than someone who doesn't drink regularly. The brain has somehow adapted to the presence of sedative drugs (such as alcohol) and this alters the response to anaesthetic drugs. Regular or heavy drinkers often require unusually large doses of anaesthetic to put them to sleep and maintain anaesthesia. This can cause some minor problems for the anaesthetist if he is not forewarned.

Heavy drinkers may present other problems. Beer drinkers may get a substantial proportion of their daily calorie intake from beer and as a consequence have a poor diet lacking in some vitamins. Any heavy drinker may suffer withdrawal symptoms with the enforced abstinence during a stay in hospital. Often this doesn't present until after an operation when the patient becomes acutely agitated, confused and may even hallucinate. Finally, heavy drinking may cause acute inflammation or cirrhosis of the liver, both of which compromise the liver's ability to break down drugs and produce important blood proteins such as clotting factors.

Surprisingly small quantities of alcohol on a regular basis can damage your health. The recommended maximum weekly intake of alcohol to avoid any damage to your health is 20 units of alcohol for men and 15 for women. One unit of alcohol is contained in half a pint of beer, a standard measure of spirits or one glass of wine. If, as a male you are drinking more than one-and-a-half pints of beer a day, you are over the limit!

MEDICATIONS

Most regular medicines should be continued up to and during the period of an operation. Certain drugs such as insulin, steroids and anticoagulants will need adjustment while you are in hospital but should be continued as normal until you are admitted to hospital. Some other drugs increase the risk of complications during the anaesthetic or operation and may need to be stopped in advance. This includes a certain type of antidepressant drug called Mono-amine Oxidase Inhibitors (MAOIs for short) which may seriously interact with the anaesthetic. If you are on this type of drug you will have been given a warning card to carry on your person in case of emergency.

A much more common drug that may need to be stopped is the birth control pill. It has been proven that the pill substantially increases the risk of deep venous thrombosis (blood clot in the legs) after any major operation. In a small proportion of cases this can lead to a potentially fatal condition known as pulmonary embolus. The blood clot becomes detached from the wall of the vein, travels through the heart and blocks blood flow to the lungs. A large clot is immediately fatal but usually, smaller clots give the warning signs of sudden, sharp chest pain and shortness of breath. Treatment is very effective if not too late. The chances of this serious complication can be reduced by stopping the pill four weeks before any major operation. Consult your doctor at an early stage and discuss alternative methods of contraception. Many minor operations carry very little risk of this complication and it is not then necessary to stop the pill. The 'mini-pill' which does not contain oestrogens does not have this hazard.

The subject of deep venous thrombosis and its prevention is important and is covered in more detail in the chapter on post-operative recovery. Many lives are tragically lost because of failure to take simple and effective precautions against this common complication.

DENTAL TREATMENT

A general anaesthetic often involves passing tubes or instruments into the mouth. If you have any loose, fragile or badly decayed teeth, these may possibly become dislodged in the course of the anaesthetic. This is a hazard because a tooth or fragment may be inhaled. Anaesthetists take a great deal of care with teeth but it is sensible to have them in good condition before an anaesthetic. The upper front teeth are most vulnerable and this applies particularly if any are capped or crowned. If you have a large and expensive row of delicate porcelain crowns that worry you, it is possible for your dentist to reinforce or protect these prior to an anaesthetic. Discuss it with your dentist. Any badly decayed teeth should be extracted before your operation.

3 Admission to Hospital

THE WAITING LIST

After your appointment in the outpatient clinic, your name is put on the waiting list for an operation. Now comes a wait which may be anything from a few days to a year or more. One paradox is that the longer you wait, the shorter the notice you are likely to get of your operation. For instance if you have waited a year for a hernia repair, the letter of invitation for your operation may only arrive two days in advance! Susan, whom we met earlier, is a highly organised sort of person, and she cannot understand this apparent lack of planning. It seems to her an example of gross inefficiency in the NHS which doesn't occur in the private hospitals. Actually, there are great difficulties in planning ahead and as the subject of waiting lists arouses so much feeling, it is worth explaining how they are operated.

Each consultant has their own waiting list and the length of this list may differ between surgeons and vary markedly between health districts. This depends on the relationship between local resources and the demand for this particular service. Each consultant is provided with a certain number of beds in the hospital – often a single ward –, a fixed number of operating sessions per week and a small team of doctors to assist him in operating, and in running the clinics and ward. The consultant is free to organise his waiting list however he likes. If the consultant dealt only with routine cases, operations could be planned well in advance to fill all the available operating sessions and use all his allocation of beds. Unfortunately, a considerable proportion of a consultant's bed-space and operating time is taken up with emergency cases which are entirely unpredictable. The different consultant surgeons in a hospital take it in turn to accept all emergency admissions for a twenty-four hour period and this occurs on several days of each week. Because of continual drives for 'efficiency', many hospitals are run with almost all the beds constantly occupied. Routine admissions often have to wait some hours for a patient to be discharged before a bed is freed for their use. Quite often, emergency admissions will use up all of a consultant's free beds and he then has to borrow bed spaces on other wards to accommodate further emergency

Admission to Hospital · 37

cases. This disrupts the organisation of routine admissions to several wards, often leading to last-minute cancellations.

So what happens is this: A relatively small number of routine, major operations need to be performed urgently. For instance, if the surgeon diagnoses bowel cancer, he will be anxious to do the operation within a few weeks. Cases such as these are given the highest priority and are booked for a certain date in advance. Because of the relatively small number involved, it is very unlikely that these operations will be postponed. Next in priority come a larger number of less urgent cases which are used to fill up the bulk of the operating time available. These are also mostly planned in advance although just how many can be fitted in will depend on day to day variations in bed availability. Finally, there are a large number of non-urgent operations such as hernia repair or removal of various benign lumps that are used as 'stocking fillers'. Some are booked onto junior surgeon's operating lists but many are arranged at very short notice to fill up any available beds or operating time when the uncertainties of that week's emergencies have revealed themselves. Surgeons will try hard to fill any unexpected gaps in their operating sessions and it is not uncommon for patients to be contacted by telephone and invited to have an operation the following day! So, please be tolerant. The hospital staff will try very hard to plan your operation in advance and they find the limited resources a continual frustration.

One partial solution to the problem of planning minor operations is to perform them as day cases in an independent unit with its own beds and operating theatres. These facilities are not used for any emergency cases and as every patient is discharged by the end of the day, all beds are always available for the following day. Efficient planning is therefore possible.

INVITATION FOR ADMISSION

When your name finally comes to the top of the waiting list, you will be invited by letter to come to hospital. It usually reads something like the one overleaf.

Read your admission letter carefully. Different versions are sent out depending on the circumstances and there may be important instructions such as: 'Take no food and drink after midnight of the day before admission'. If these instructions are ignored your operation may be cancelled. Also read the accompanying booklets or sheets. These give much useful information and explanation. My own hospital sends out the following with the admission letter:

- A health questionnaire for the patient to complete and bring with them.

38 · Admission to Hospital

Tel:430014 Ext 4308
                                                     Admissions Unit
Medical Records Department
Eastern Infirmary
West Street
Bigtown

Susan Williams   16 November 1988
12 Horton Drive
Hillswood   Ref: 638277
Bigtown

Dear Mrs Williams,

A bed has been reserved for you at the Eastern Infirmary, please see details below:

Consultant : Mr Brown
Speciality : General surgery
Admission date : 10 May 1989
Ward : Ward 11
Time : 2.30pm

Please ring the above ward on the morning of admission to confirm that your bed is still available and on arrival report to Reception in the main corridor of the hospital.

Ambulance transport has not been arranged for you. However, if you think an ambulance is necessary on medical grounds, please consult your family doctor.

If you cannot come to hospital on the date given, please inform the Admissions Unit, Ext 4308 as soon as possible so that your bed may be offered to another patient.

Please read carefully the enclosed booklet.

MEDICINES It is very important that you take the enclosed leaflet concerning medicines and drugs to your family doctor for completion.

Yours sincerely,

Medical Records Manager.

Admission to Hospital · 39

- A form for the family doctor to complete about drug treatment.
- A general information and advice booklet about your hospital stay.
- Advice on the hospital no-smoking policy.
- Instructions about hospital meals and menu cards.

If you live on your own you will have to remember to make your house secure and cancel deliveries of milk and newspapers. It may be sensible to turn off the gas, electricity or water or to ask a neighbour to keep an eye on the house. If you have a state pension or any other benefit, you should tell the local DHSS when you are going into hospital. If you have difficulties or worries about these, the hospital social worker will be able to help or advise you when you are in hospital.

WHAT TO TAKE TO HOSPITAL?

What personal items should you bring? I suggest the following items:

Nightdress or pyjamas
Underwear
Dressing gown
Slippers
Personal toiletry items (incl razor for the men)
Paper tissues
Pen, paper and reading material
Reading glasses
Small change for the telephone, papers and items from the hospital shop trolley
The name, address and telephone numbers of next of kin and of friends or neighbours if they are helping with your journey home from hospital

Pyjamas

A word of advice that may surprise the ladies: If you are having a major operation, especially an abdominal operation, consider wearing pyjamas in hospital rather than a nightdress. The reason is this. After an operation, the doctors on the ward will want to keep an eye on your tummy and listen to your chest quite often. If you are wearing a nightdress, this will have to be lifted up above your waist every time. When you have a painful abdominal wound after an operation, this may become quite an ordeal, lifting your bottom and struggling to shift your night clothes up and down. Pyjamas make this infinitely easier and more comfortable and also provide more decent cover in what is a fairly public place.

MEDICINES

It is very important to bring with you any medicines or tablets you are taking at home. Although your family doctor will have been asked to provide this information, it is surprising how often their records of prescriptions are out of date. You will be asked to hand in your tablets and medicines when you are admitted to the ward and some hospitals do not return them to the patients on discharge. I think this is unfair, particularly if you have paid for the prescription. If you are on long-term treatment that will be continued after your hospital stay, take in only one packet or label for each of your medicines. Your prescriptions may be changed on discharge and the ward doctor will write a note for your family doctor with these details.

TRANSPORT TO HOSPITAL

You are expected to make your own way to hospital, either by public transport, or with the help of family or friends. Driving yourself to hospital is rarely practical as you may not be in a fit state to drive on discharge. Besides, finding a park may be difficult and your car will not be secure left unguarded for days and nights.

If you are ill, or disabled, or are elderly without anyone to help, then ambulance transport can be provided although this must be arranged in advance. This is sometimes arranged at the time of your outpatient visit. Otherwise, you must read carefully the instructions on the invitation to admission. Some hospitals will ask you to contact your family doctor. Others will ask you to ring the hospital admissions department in advance. Like all other resources in the NHS, ambulances are in short supply and efficient use is made by booking in advance. Except in an emergency, you cannot arrange an ambulance without one or two days advanced notice. Arrangements for your transport home will be made by the hospital staff, if necessary.

THE ADMISSION PROCEDURE

On arrival at the hospital, report to the admissions office. This will be close to the main entrance of the hospital and should be well signposted. The hospital admissions or reception office functions in exactly the same way as a hotel reception. Patients are identified, registered, and allocated a bed on a ward. The admissions staff keep track of empty beds in the hospital on an hour-to-hour basis and allocate patients accordingly. This is a complex and difficult task because of all the uncertainties in the demand and supply of beds, most of which are occupied. Not only do the staff have to deal with large numbers of patients being admitted at reception but they also have to liaise with the on-call doctors who need beds for emergency cases. On busy days, the situation changes hour by hour and there is a constant stream of telephone calls, cancellations, negotiations, apologies and last minute changes. Sometimes, patients are 'phoned at home or work and asked to come in at very short notice if unexpected vacancies occur. This is a thankless task carried out with mostly good humour and tact, twenty-four hours a day. Personally, I admire the admissions staff and wouldn't do their job for anything! So, if you are kept waiting, please try to understand and be patient even though you may be feeling very nervous and anxious about the uncertainties of your operation and hospital stay. Have a chat with your neighbour in the waiting room; you'll find plenty in common. Perhaps you are going to the same ward.

When you are registered, the admissions officer will confirm your name, address, date of birth and the name and address of your family doctor. If any of these details have changed, make sure that they have the up-to-date version. You will be asked for the name, address and telephone number of your next of kin, for your occupation and religion. If you are not of British nationality, the length of your stay in the UK will be asked as this may affect your entitlement to free treatment under the NHS.

You may then be asked to wait until your bed is available on the ward. Alternatively, you may be shown to the ward straight away, either to your bed, or to wait in the ward day-room. In some hospitals you may be directed to the x-ray department or pathology clinic to have tests done while you wait. This will save time for the doctor on the ward and at least occupies some of your waiting time usefully.

When you reach the ward, you should identify yourself to one of the nurses or the ward receptionist. You won't be sent to the ward until you are expected, so don't hesitate to walk onto the ward. Often you will find a nurse at a desk half way along the ward, or else in an office at the side.

When you are shown to your bed, you will be asked to change into your night clothes in preparation for examination by the ward doctor. This is the moment when you may begin to feel the loss of identity, privacy and dignity inherent in a stay in hospital. To the hospital staff this is probably just a matter of routine but I can remember how self conscious, embarrassed and demeaned I felt, having to change into pyjamas in a public place in the middle of the day. The only consolation is that everyone else is in the same boat.

Your bed will be shielded from the rest of the ward by curtains which, unlike a door, no one can knock at to ask to come in. Not infrequently, a doctor may suddenly step through the curtains when you are half undressed and you may find this embarrassing, especially if you are of the opposite sex. With any luck, you will be able to complete changing and establish your territory with the curtains pulled back before anyone approaches. You are provided with a bedside locker in which to store your personal belongings and a few clothes. If you have any valuable possessions or excess money with you, these should be locked up in the hospital safe and a receipt will be given to you. The bed-side locker is not a secure place for valuables.

ADMISSION BY A NURSE

The admission process on the ward takes place in two stages with a certain amount of repetition. You are usually seen first by a nurse, and later by the houseman (ward doctor), who will each question you and make notes. Often you will be seen by a pupil nurse. Enquiries will be made about all your personal habits such as diet, sleeping, bowel action and so on which the nursing staff will use as a guide to your post-operative care. The nurse may also request details of your past medical history. You will be asked again for the name, address and telephone number of your next of kin or whoever else you would like contacted in case of difficulty or changed arrangements.

You will be shown a plastic identity bracelet and asked to confirm the details of your name and date of birth. This bracelet also shows your hospital records number. This number is unique to you and if you attend the same hospital again, you will still have the same number. This number is recorded on all your notes, specimens, x-rays and laboratory reports as a check of identity. This bracelet will be attached to your wrist or ankle and should not be removed until you are discharged from hospital. It is your safeguard against mistaken identity to prevent confusion over diagnosis or which operation you are having. It is surprisingly common to find patients with the same surname on the ward simultaneously. The nurse will label the head of the bed with your own name, and the name of the consultant whose care you are under.

You will be weighed, asked for a specimen of urine, and will have your pulse rate, blood pressure and temperature recorded on a chart at the end of your bed. If you have any particular worries or queries about day-to-day matters, ask the nurse. She will probably be able to put your mind at rest and can write a memo in the notes if necessary.

If you have brought any medicines or tablets with you, these should be collected together and surrendered to either the nurse or doctor. You must not take any of your own tablets during your stay in hospital as these might seriously interfere with your treatment. If you need to continue tablets, the houseman will prescribe them for administration by the nursing staff. Careful records are made of every tablet or medicine given.

Admission to Hospital · 43

CLERKING BY THE DOCTOR

The next person to see you will be the houseman. This is the most junior doctor on the surgeon's team, and the one you will see most often. A description of the houseman's job and responsibilities is given in the chapter on hospital staff.

He or she will 'clerk' you. This means asking a lot of questions, examining you, and often doing some blood tests and other special tests. This can take anything from ten minutes to well over an hour. The doctor will ask you about the following:

- The symptoms of your surgical condition and how they developed. If you have been on the waiting list a long time, these might have changed or improved so it is important to go into these details again in case a different treatment is needed
- Questions about your general health, often known as a 'review of the systems'. This includes enquiry about your heart and circulation, breathing, eating and bowel habits, bladder function, sleeping, and any neurological problems. These questions are designed to assess your general health and to discover any symptoms that you might not have thought important to mention
- Past history of illness or operations
- What medications you are taking, and any known allergies
- Your smoking and drinking habits
- Any significant illness that runs in the family, the 'family history'. You will be asked if your parents are still alive, and if not, how they died
- Your occupation and social circumstances. If you are elderly and live alone, enquiry will be made into which social services you receive or may need after your operation, such as meals-on-wheels or home help

Next comes the physical examination. This is in two parts, firstly to detect signs of your surgical condition and secondly to assess your fitness for the operation and anaesthetic. The doctor will feel and count your pulse, count your rate of breathing and measure your blood pressure. He will check the colour of your skin, the white of your eyes, and the pinkness of the inside of your eyelids. This is to detect any signs of jaundice or anaemia. If it is relevant, he may feel for enlarged glands in the neck, under the arms and in the groins. He will look in your mouth.

The chest is examined by tapping with a finger to check the drum-like resonance, feeling for chest expansion, and listening to breath sounds with a stethoscope. The heart is examined by feeling for the position of the heart beat on the left side of the chest and by listening to the heart sounds and any extra sounds such as a heart murmur.

The abdomen is examined in a similar manner by tapping, feeling and listening. The groins will be examined especially carefully if you have a hernia. The legs will be examined carefully if you have varicose veins, ulcers, deformed toes or any other surgical condition of the legs.

In some patients, particularly those having an abdominal operation or women having an operation on the womb or vagina, it may be necessary to do an internal examination. This is dreaded by many people but it need not be any worse than a little uncomfortable and embarrassing.

Rectal examination (the back passage) allows the doctor to diagnose or exclude several important conditions. These include cancer of the rectum, inflammatory swellings or abscesses, enlargement of the prostate gland in men, and some types of internal cancer in women. No doctor likes performing rectal examination and it is usually done in the middle-aged or older patient who may be at risk of these conditions.

Here's how it is done. Patients are asked to pull down their pants and lie on their left side with the knees drawn up towards the chest. The doctor will wear thin plastic or rubber gloves. A small amount of lubricating jelly is placed at the back passage and this often feels cold. The doctor will then ask you to relax your back passage – naturally tensed at this moment – and will very gently insert just a single finger. Unless you have a tender condition such as an anal fissure, this will not be at all painful. Some people get in a panic because they feel as if they are passing stool but this is just the natural sensation of the anus being distended. Don't worry, it's almost impossible to soil yourself in the circumstances. The doctor will need to feel around in all directions and mostly all you can feel is pushing at the back passage. There are, however, two sensitive areas, one in men and one in women. In men, the prostate gland, which lies just under the neck of the bladder, is just in front of the rectum. The doctor will feel this carefully with the fingertip and this can be rather a startling sensation if you weren't expecting it, but not painful. In women, the vagina lies immediately in front of the rectum and the doctor will be able to feel the cervix as a lump at the end of the vagina. This may cause a funny 'inside' sensation which is not painful either. When the doctor has finished, he will wipe your bottom although it may still feel rather slimy from the jelly.

Examination of the front passage in women can be done in the same position, or with the patient lying on their back with knees drawn up and apart. As before, lubricating gel and gloves are used and usually two fingers are gently inserted. Often, the doctor will feel in the lower abdomen at the same time so that he can judge the size of the womb or other swellings by feeling between his two hands. If the doctor requires a clear view of the

Admission to Hospital · 45

cervix, a spoon-shaped instrument called a speculum will be gently inserted to hold open the vaginal walls. Examination of the front passage is done most frequently on the gynaecological wards which specialise in women's complaints. It is not performed very often on the general surgical ward.

The rank of houseman now contains almost equal numbers of men and women so you are quite likely to be seen by a doctor of opposite sex. When doctors are faced with young patients of the opposite sex, they will be sensitive to the feelings of embarrassment of the patient and may also be afraid of accusations of molesting or indecent assault. For this reason, it is customary for the doctor to have a nurse present to act as chaperon in these circumstances.

If you are a fit, young person having a minor operation, you probably won't require any tests and the clerking procedure will be finished. If, like George, you are older and having a major operation, a whole battery of tests will be done, both as an aid to diagnosis and to assess your fitness for the operation and anaesthetic. Blood samples for testing are usually taken on the ward but for most other investigations, you will be taken to another part of the hospital. The chapter on tests and investigations describes what these are for and how they are done. If you are having any blood tests done, the houseman will probably take a sample when he has finished examining you. Finally, the houseman will ask you to sign a form consenting to operation. The subject of consent to operation is so important that I have devoted a whole chapter to the subject. Don't sign the form until you have read the chapter!

You will probably now be left to your own devices. Both the nurses and doctors will be very busy admitting other patients and this is your chance to explore your new surroundings. Do not leave the ward unless you have first checked with one of the nurses. You may be required for further tests, and later in the day, one of the more senior surgeons will want to see you before your operation. This will usually be a very brief visit with perhaps examination of the part to be operated on. You should make the most of this single opportunity to discuss your operation in detail with the surgeon who will actually perform it. The houseman may be relatively ignorant of the details of your treatment. Don't be afraid to ask questions. Often this visit will take place in the late afternoon or early evening when the surgeon has finished the rest of his day's work.

If you are needed for tests such as x-rays outside the ward, then a hospital porter will come and fetch you with a wheelchair. This insistence on the use of a wheelchair reinforces your role as a helpless patient even if you are perfectly capable of walking. This has to be borne with as much dignity as you can muster as argument is useless. It is almost impossible to bend the rules which aim to make you completely passive and incapable of independent action. The reliance on wheelchairs also means that you may be faced with a long wait for your journey back to the ward while the porter is busy elsewhere. Never mind! Strike up a conversation with someone else in the waiting room and time will pass more quickly.

LIFE ON THE WARD

An old-fashioned ward will have changed little since Florence Nightingale's time. A single large room may have twenty or thirty beds ranked along the two walls, with a common space in-between. Many NHS hospitals are like this. Wards designed more recently will be sub-divided into smaller rooms or bays and these will afford better privacy. You may even have the privacy of a single room but this has some disadvantages including lack of company except during the restricted visiting hours. Also, after your operation, the nursing staff will not be able to observe you as closely as a patient on the main ward.

Beside your bed you will have a locker and a chair. The extent of your territory is marked by curtains that hang from a rail and your nearest neighbour will not be many feet away. On the wall behind your bed there will be a lamp, oxygen supply and a suction device. A handset on the end of a cable will have buttons to control the light and to call a nurse. Earphones are usually available, tuned to a selection of radio stations.

Most surgical wards are single sex but some have both sexes, separated only by a partition half way along the ward. If the sexes are mixed, there will be separate bathrooms at each end of the ward. Bathroom facilities are often limited and will be especially crowded in the early mornings. If you want to have a bath, this is often easier during the day.

Every ward will have a day room with easy chairs, a television and a selection of books and magazines. Smoking is not permitted on the ward, in the bathroom or in the day room. If you cannot survive without smoking, ask one of the nurses who will tell you where you can go outside the ward. Admission to hospital is a good opportunity to give up smoking and I have already discussed the benefits of this for your post-operative recovery.

The ward day tends to start rather early and often the nurses will make their first round with the drugs trolley at six o'clock in the morning. Breakfast will be served before eight o'clock and is taken at tables in the centre of the ward like the other meals unless you are bed bound. On some mornings of the week, the consultant will do his ward-round and the nursing staff will be particularly anxious to have the ward tidy and regimented before he arrives. Visitors are rarely allowed in the morning but the ward will be open for a couple of hours in the mid afternoon and also in the evening. Most wards restrict the number of your visitors to two at any one time. If you feel too tired or ill to receive many visitors, tell one of the nurses and visitors will be restricted on 'doctors orders'. This will not cause any offence and it is important that you have the rest you need.

At regular intervals during the day and evening, a trolley will tour the ward offering hot drinks. Sometimes, the fitter patients give a help with this task. You are provided with a glass and jug of water on your locker and it is handy to have a bottle of squash to flavour this. The wards tend to be rather warm and you will become thirsty without regular drinks.

During the day, the hospital shop will visit the ward with a large trolley heaped with goodies. This includes confectionary, biscuits and snacks, drinks, toiletry items and a small selection of reading matter. A newsagent will call with the daily papers. Every hospital has a lending library and often a selection is brought round the wards if you are not able to visit the library yourself.

A telephone trolley is usually available to make outside calls from the bedside.

Patients choose their meals a day in advance by filling in a menu card on the ward. This gives a limited choice but arrangements are made for patients with special dietry needs, because of religion or medical condition.

Ward rounds

Doctors will do various sorts of ward rounds. Every day, several of the doctors will do a quick 'business round' in which the care and progress of all the patients will be reviewed. Charts will be examined, wounds inspected and brief enquiry made. This is conducted very briskly and decisions about drips, tubes, drinking, eating etc are made. Often this will take place twice a day.

Each consultant will hold a formal ward round, usually once or twice a week. This may take some hours and is often preceded by a meeting in the office where notes are reviewed. The entire team of surgeons will be present, accompanied by the nursing sister and sometimes other members of staff. The consultant will probably take the opportunity to teach his more junior colleagues and so the history of a few patients will be related in detail and discussed at the end of the bed. Don't be alarmed if this happens to you. It's not a reflection of the severity of your illness but just an indication that your case is interesting and informative for the junior doctors. Not all the remarks will apply to you as the condition may be discussed in general, including various forms of treatment. Few patients are singled out in this way on the ward round as most will already have had their operations. Often there's just a brief 'how-do-you-do' which may be the only contact you ever have with your consultant.

The third type of ward round is a teaching round for the benefit of student doctors. This only occurs in the teaching hospitals, usually in the larger cities. The round is conducted by the consultant or senior registrar accompanied by up to eight student doctors. You will not be chosen as a subject unless you have previously given your permission. One of the students will have clerked you in the same manner as the houseman and will be expected to make a formal presentation of your history and examination at the bedside. I remember this as a considerable ordeal when I was a student as the opportunities for humiliation and embarrassment were plentiful and enjoyed by some of the senior surgeons. It can be quite interesting hearing your case discussed with the medical students as this will be at an elementary level, more comprehensible than the jargon of the business rounds. Often another student will be asked to demonstrate their examination technique in front of the audience. If you have a clear physical sign such as a lump or swelling, your permission may be sought for everyone to have a feel of it.

THE EVE OF YOUR OPERATION

The evening before surgery, the early preparations will begin. You will be starved at least six hours before any anaesthetic and if you are on the morning operation list, you will not be allowed to eat or drink anything after midnight. A notice will be placed on your bed, NIL BY MOUTH AFTER MIDNIGHT. Often the site of operation will be shaved. This is done either by a hospital barber, or one of the ward staff. The site of operation will be marked with ink so there can be no mistake about which side is to be operated on. The exact course of varicose veins will be marked as these disappear when you are lying down. Small, mobile lumps that are hard to feel are marked accurately otherwise you may just have a crude arrow which indicates the general area of surgery. The mark will be made either by the houseman or the surgeon who will perform the operation. Sometimes, no mark will be made. For instance it's not possible to take out the wrong gall-bladder, you only have one! If you have a mark, do not wash it off.

The early morning start on the ward is followed by early bed-time and often the ward lights will be turned out soon after ten at night. If you wish to read later, you can use the lamp by your bed. It can be hard to sleep on your first night in hospital with the worry of an operation the next day. Also the ward may be quite busy and noisy at night with various disturbances including emergency admissions. A good night's sleep is important so it is worth considering a sleeping pill. Despite the bad reputation of sleeping pills, the modern drugs will send you to sleep and then wear off in a few hours, leaving no hangover effects. They are not in any way addictive taken over a short period, so I would recommend a pill if you do have trouble sleeping. The same sort of pill may well be used for your premedication before anaesthesia.

Anaesthetist's visit

Most anaesthetists will visit their patients on the ward before surgery. For a morning operation, visits are often made in the evening before, at the end of a day's work. It is the responsibility of the anaesthetist to decide if you are fit for surgery and anaesthesia, and cases are sometimes postponed if the anaesthetist thinks that the patient's condition could be improved with further treatment. For instance, if a patient's blood pressure was very high, new treatment would be started to control the blood pressure before the anaesthetic to avoid unnecessary risk. The anaesthetist will study the notes the houseman has made and look at the results of blood tests or x-rays.

He will then come and talk to you about the anaesthetic and pain relief after the operation. He may want to enquire more closely about your general health and will inspect your teeth, mouth and neck to anticipate any technical difficulties with the anaesthetic. You should tell him about any capped or crowned teeth but ordinary fillings are not of concern.

Many patients worry more about the anaesthetic than the surgery. Apart from reassurance, the anaesthetist may be able to offer an alternative form of anaesthesia if you have a particular dread of general anaesthetics. Often patients have had bad experiences in the past but the modern anaesthetist will be able to avoid many of these problems with improved techniques or drugs. He will ask if you want a pre-med tablet or injection to reduce anxiety and may prescribe other forms of treatment with the pre-med.

DAY-CASE SURGERY

There is an increasing vogue for performing minor surgery in specialised day case units which can be run more efficiently and economically than general surgical wards. By avoiding an overnight stay, considerable savings are made and there is less disruption of patient's work or family life.

The ward and operating theatre are staffed only during the day and all patients have their operation and go home on the same day. Usually patients are asked to report to the day theatre reception and not to the main hospital reception. The whole procedure is streamlined and carefully planned. Only fit patients having minor surgery are listed and they are assessed in advance, in the outpatient clinic. Instructions must be followed carefully, or your operation may be postponed.

Patients for morning surgery are asked to report at seven-thirty or eight o'clock in the morning with instructions not to drink or eat anything after midnight. You are asked to change into a hospital gown and will be seen briefly by the surgeon and anaesthetist before the list begins. A varying proportion of the cases are done under local anaesthetic.

After a short rest, your recovery from the anaesthetic will be assessed and

50 · Admission to Hospital

once you are clear headed and steady on your feet, you will be allowed home. Patients who have had a general anaesthetic are not permitted to travel alone and your operation won't be done unless you have someone to accompany you on the journey and at home afterwards. You must not drive until the following day. Although the anaesthetist will choose drugs that are rapidly cleared from the body, you may still experience a slight hangover effect with drowsiness or poor concentration for the rest of the day.

Morning patients are usually discharged by early afternoon, at the latest, to make room for the afternoon list.

4 The Hospital Staff

'Your life in their hands' was the apt name of a television documentary series about the dramas of hospital practice. The title acknowledged the teamwork involved in the care of each patient. Writing this chapter reminded me just how remarkable a team of professionals is involved, and I was impressed by the enormous investment in training and qualifications of the large team involved with each patient. Perhaps twenty or thirty staff will be directly involved in your care. Some you will meet and some, like the laboratory staff, remain in the background performing equally important tasks.

This chapter is about the staff you will meet, who they are and what they do. Over many years, a comprehensive system of care has developed in which different aspects of your treatment are managed by professionals with specialised training. This means that responsibility for your care is divided amongst many different staff who then work together as a team. Unless you understand the roles of the different staff, your stay in hospital can be a bewildering experience and you will find it difficult to contribute to your treatment and recovery.

Understanding who the different staff are will make life much easier on the ward and you will be able to appreciate how all the different aspects of your therapy fit together like the pieces of a jig saw. Hospital patients often find it very difficult to communicate with the staff because they direct their questions to the wrong person. They are then frustrated by an inadequate or ill informed answer, or else directed to question another member of staff they don't recognise. Many of the hospital staff are distinguished by different uniforms and I will describe these for each member of the team so that you can recognise them.

It is hard to remember the details of all the staff but you will find this chapter a valuable reference once you are in hospital and have met some of the team.

DOCTORS

In the course of your hospital stay you are likely to meet a number of doctors who play different roles. One will be the anaesthetist and others will be members of the surgical team who work together under the supervision of your consultant. It is helpful to understand the rank and titles of the different doctors, and what their jobs are.

The full surgical team comprises the consultant, senior registrar, registrar, senior house officer and house officer (otherwise known as the houseman). These are ranked in descending order of seniority and experience. This team is known as a 'firm' but it is rare to have the full complement of doctors except in some of the large teaching hospitals. Usually, one or two of the intermediate grades are left out or shared between consultants.

The houseman

The doctor you will see most is the houseman. In recent years, almost half of the graduates from medical schools have been female so you are quite likely to have a female houseman. For the sake of simplicity I will refer to the houseman as 'he', without any slight intended towards the equally competent women doctors.

The houseman is the doctor who first sees you when you arrive on the ward and it is his responsibility to make sure you are fit for the anaesthetic and surgery by recording your history and performing a physical examination. The houseman is also responsible for looking after you on the ward after your operation where you will see him daily.

The houseman is in his first year of training after qualification and every doctor, whether they want to be a GP or hospital specialist, has to do this job for six months. This first year is the hardest of any doctor's career and the job often borders on the impossible. The houseman is general dogsbody on the firm and has an enormous load of routine work: clerking the new patients, doing or arranging large numbers of tests, arranging the operating lists, caring for all the patients post-operatively, writing all the notes and prescription charts, and pandering to the whims of the consultant. He is expected to know the details of all the patients and present them on the consultant's ward round. He is also expected to assist in the operating theatre. He acts as liaison between all the different staff connected with a patient's care and generally ensures that everything runs smoothly despite a hundred and one conflicting requirements.

But in addition, he will be rostered on call for emergency duties and ward work at night without any relief from his routine duties. Thus, several days each week and commonly at weekends, he will be required to work all day, all night and all the next day, sometimes without any sleep at all. On the worst sort of day, he might be occupied all morning with a ward round, have seven routine admissions to clerk in the afternoon and at the same time have to deal with ten or twenty emergency admissions, sometimes very seriously ill. He is slave to his bleep which interrupts his work, demanding immediate attention to calls from within and outside the hospital. A single weekend shift will sometimes last from Friday morning until Monday evening. To add insult to injury, the fifty or more hours of overtime in a week are paid at only one third of the basic rate.

So, if at times the houseman appears zombie like, dishevelled, inattentive, surly, rude or insensitive it's probably because he's been working flat out for 36 hours or more without any sleep. Have sympathy, because the quality of your care depends to quite an extent on the houseman. The good houseman will act as your ambassador and will constantly represent your interests so that you get swift and expert attention. A well organised houseman will have built up contacts in all the various hospital departments and will, for instance, be able to organise x-rays and other tests for you more quickly than if he used the usual channels. If you have any queries or special requests, he can present these to the more senior staff. Finally, if he has a good working relationship with the nursing staff on the ward, they are more likely to take extra trouble with your own care.

The houseman will see you daily and check on your progress. He will also perform a variety of minor practical procedures such as replacing an intravenous drip.

The Senior House Officer (SHO)

This is the next most senior doctor on the firm who will have been qualified for between one and five years. Many SHOs have chosen to follow a career in surgery although some will be gaining extra hospital experience before becoming a GP. Early in their career, they will learn to perform operations under close supervision but as their experience broadens, they will be allowed to do first minor, and then more major, surgery on their own, with help if need be. A lot of their experience comes from doing emergency cases at night. It is quite possible that your own operation will be performed by the SHO and if this is the case, he will be sure to see you on the ward before your operation, and to examine you himself. The SHO is responsible for supervising the houseman and the two will work closely together, especially on the days and nights when they accept emergency patients. The SHO will also assist the consultant in the outpatient clinics and you may already have met him there. The SHO works just as long hours as the houseman but is generally spared all the dogsbody work of the houseman and usually gets more sleep. However, in some jobs, particularly in the surgical specialities such as gynaecology or orthopaedics, there may not be a houseman on the firm and then the SHO has effectively to do both jobs.

What little spare time the SHO has will be spent studying for exams such as the diploma of Fellowship of the Royal College of Surgeons. These are difficult exams without which it is impossible to progress up the career ladder.

The Registrar and Senior Registrar

Usually, there is just one surgeon of these ranks on the firm. A registrar will have been training as a surgeon for at least two or three years and often much longer. He will hold the Fellowship and will be competent to perform much of the day to day surgery, while assisting his consultant with the more major or difficult cases. The senior registrar has almost completed his professional training and is waiting for a consultant post. Because of intense competition for these posts, some senior registrars get stuck in the grade for many years and will be very experienced and skilful surgeons, more than qualified to hold a consultant's post. Like the junior doctors on the firm, the registrar or senior registrar will be on call for emergency duties several nights a week. However, the SHO will be able to deal with most of the emergency cases and so the registrar will be on call from home for the more difficult work.

Usually, the registrar (or senior registrar) will do a quick ward round with the houseman and SHO at the start of every day before the operating list begins. He will spend most of his time either in the operating theatre, doing his own list, or in the outpatient clinic. He will join the rest of the firm for the consultant's ward round. Often he will have research interests and he may be working towards a higher degree. He will also help with the administration of the firm and will often attend scientific meetings with other doctors or give lectures himself.

The Consultant

The consultants are kings of the hospital and have a great deal of autonomy. They are employed at a regional level so, at present, the district health authority in which they work has a limited influence on the terms of their contract. This situation is changing with recent government reforms of the NHS. They are contracted to work a certain number of hours within the NHS and this leaves a small amount of time to do private practice if they so wish. In fact most consultant surgeons work extremely hard and devote many more hours to their NHS work than their contract demands. Each consultant is ultimately responsible for the care of patients under his name. This includes responsibility for the work of all members of his firm and ensuring adequate training and supervision of his junior staff. Within the limitations of the available resources (beds, operating sessions, clinics, staff) he must try and meet the demands for both emergency and planned surgery but otherwise he may run the service as he sees fit.

Until recently there were no financial limitations on his work and almost no attempt to measure the quality or 'efficiency' of his service. This has changed drastically in recent years with the introduction of very strict limits on hospital spending in the face of ever increasing demand for ever more expensive treatment. Consultants now have a much greater responsibility for the financial budgets of their department and many are now auditing the work of their firm with careful record keeping and analysis, often with the aid of computers. This includes such measures as the number of operations performed, the average length of hospital stay, and the rate of complications or death.

So far, consultants have retained the right to make clinical decisions about a patient's treatment free from any managerial restraint. This is a very important safeguard because the best interests of the patient are served without any financial, social or political control being exerted. Consultants tend to develop their own individual style and values and practice does vary significantly between consultants treating even the same condition. In a sense, this gives the patient a certain choice as the family doctor has the right to choose any consultant in the health district, and sometimes beyond.

Consultants wield considerable power over the junior doctors who cannot hope to progress up the career ladder without their support. In the first few years of a doctor's career, contracts are only granted for six month periods. This means that junior doctors are constantly searching for the next job. The appointment of doctors right up to the senior registrar level is made by consultants and no one is appointed unless they have good references from their previous consultants. There is very stiff competition for posts in the major hospitals and, especially here, the junior doctors will try very hard to impress their consultants. Some of the older consultants, especially, enjoy this position and like to display their rank on the weekly ward rounds. Many other consultants are much more informal and sympathetic towards their junior staff.

It is quite possible that you may never meet your consultant, either in the clinic or during your hospital stay. A substantial proportion of the work on the firm is done by the registrar or senior registrar and the consultant will ensure that this is to a standard that matches his own. Consultants hold ward rounds once or twice a week and if you are on the ward that day, you will meet the consultant even if only for brief social greetings and enquiry about your progress.

Consultant surgeons often specialise in one of the various types of surgery. These include gynaecology (women's organs), orthopaedics (bone and joint), ear nose and throat, chest surgery, plastic surgery, vascular surgery (arteries), heart surgery, ophthalmology (eyes), paediatrics (babies and children), urology (waterworks), neurosurgery (brain and nerves) and finally, general surgery which covers all the rest including abdominal surgery. Often general surgeons will have a special interest and experience in one of the more specialised fields. After qualifying, a surgeon will work and train for between ten and fifteen years before becoming a consultant. He usually then holds that post until retirement.

The anaesthetist

The anaesthetist is the doctor who will administer the anaesthetic and carefully watch over you for every minute of the operation until you have recovered from the anaesthetic. Like a surgeon, the anaesthetist is a hospital specialist who undergoes many years of training before becoming a consultant. Also, like the surgeons, there are anaesthetists of all grades from senior house officer upwards, reflecting their extent of training and experience. Similarly, they have a diploma of Fellowship of the College of Anaesthetists which co-resides with the Royal College of Surgeons in London.

In general, if you are having a minor operation, it is likely to be performed by one of the more junior surgeons working together with a junior anaesthetist. This is not grounds for concern because the new anaesthetist will not be permitted to administer any solo anaesthetic until he is trained to a competent standard. Even then, he will have expert help immediately to hand should he experience any difficulty. If an elderly or sick patient is having even only a minor operation, then a junior anaesthetist would be supervised.

Nowadays, anaesthetists offer a very wide range of services including intensive care, chronic pain relief, and pain relief in childbirth, as well as providing anaesthesia for surgery. In the intensive care unit, they look after critically ill patients for which they need a wide knowledge of medicine and pharmacology, in addition to many technical skills. Some anaesthetists specialise in anaesthesia for heart or brain surgery or one of the other surgical specialities mentioned above. Some anaesthetists are involved in research and many of the spectacular advances in surgery have come through advances in anaesthetic technique such as heart bypass. Anaesthetists are also greatly involved in the provision and training of emergency 'crash' teams who can respond within minutes to any sudden grave emergency such as cardiac arrest.

Your anaesthetist will most likely come and see you in the ward on the evening or morning before your surgery. Taking into account your level of fitness, the operation that is to be performed and a variety of other personal features, he will design an anaesthetic to suit you best.

You will next see him in the anaesthetic room which is next door to the operating theatre. By this time you may be feeling sleepy from the pre-med. When you are asleep you will be transferred into the operating theatre and, after your operation, into the recovery ward. The anaesthetist will accompany you for the whole process and will be constantly keeping watch and adjusting the anaesthetic as the operation proceeds. You will be attached to various monitors to record your pulse and blood pressure and sometimes many other measures of your well being. For a major or complicated operation, you may have more than one anaesthetist.

After the operation, the anaesthetist will make sure that you are recovering from the anaesthetic and that all your vital signs are stable. When he is satisfied, he will hand over your care to a nurse in the recovery ward who will not leave your side until you are awake. The anaesthetist is responsible for prescribing pain killers after your operation and after a major procedure will supervise your care on the ward, either directly, or by instruction to the houseman.

The radiologist

This is one other doctor you may meet. He specialises in the use of x-rays, ultrasound scanners and other devices for imaging the internal organs of the body. Although most plain x-rays are performed by radiographers, the more complex procedures may be done by the radiologist. He is also responsible for interpreting and reporting all x-ray films and related investigations.

Anyone listening to the news will be aware that an increasing number of conditions like kidney stones are now being treated without conventional surgery. Shock wave machines can focus high energy sound waves and gradually shatter stones with repeated blows. Specialised telescopes that can reach an organ through a small incision in the skin allow manipulations that would otherwise require an open operation. X-rays are used to guide these machines and so radiologists are increasingly involved in the direct treatment of patients and not just in diagnosis.

The physician

Physicians are doctors who treat patients by non-surgical means, for instance with conditions of the heart, lungs, or nervous system. Like surgeons, they can be of any rank between houseman and consultant. Physicians are not routinely involved in the care of surgical patients but occasionally advise on medical treatment of patients having surgery. If you already have a serious medical condition and are under the care of a hospital physician, then your care will be shared by the surgeon and physician.

Like surgeons, physicians tend to specialise in one field such as cardiology (heart), dermatology (skin), rheumatology (joints and arthritis) and so on.

The oncologist

This is a doctor who specialises in the treatment of cancer by non-surgical means. He can offer a wide range of treatment with drugs and x-rays. About 30% of all cancers are now cured and the oncologist can also do much to prolong life and improve its quality for those who are beyond cure. Many cancers are treated by surgery alone, in which case the oncologist wouldn't be involved. Others are treated with a combination of surgery with chemotherapy or radiotherapy and the oncologist will plan care together with the surgeon.

NURSES

British nurses are admired the world over for their compassion and professionalism. Despite this, nurses feel they do not have proper recognition of their professional status and so are revolutionizing nurse education, under the banner of 'Project 2000'. Training is being moved out of hospital into nursing schools or colleges with a greater emphasis on academic achievement and less time spent on the wards. At present, pupil nurses have a major service commitment and are paid a salary for working in the hospitals alongside qualified staff. Under Project 2000, trainees would have student status, would be paid a grant rather than a salary, and would be supernumary to the nursing establishment, although practical training would still take place on the wards.

Until now, nurses could qualify in either of two levels, as a registered nurse after a three year course, or as enrolled nurse after a more practical two year course with less stringent entry qualifications. These two levels are to be swept away and replaced with a single level of registered practitioner, a more advanced grade of specialist practitioner, and a support worker, the helper. Present enrolled nurses would be offered the chance of conversion courses to bring them up to the registered practitioner grade.

The first new courses started in 1989 with graduation after three years. For some years to come, the old grades of nurses are likely to persist and I will describe these now. Not all nurses are women, these days, so don't be surprised to find men doing the same job.

Staff nurse (Registered general nurse)
This is the largest and most highly trained group of general ward nurses. They carry a great deal of responsibility and will often be in charge of a ward, especially at night. They are responsible for the nursing care of patients, administration of drugs, the operation of medical equipment and they also have administrative duties. Staff nurses can progress up a career ladder through the grades of sister and nursing officer. Some specialise in intensive care, and some follow a longer training course in paediatric nursing (looking after children) which gives them an additional qualification.

With the limitations on NHS spending, many wards are relatively short staffed and like all grades of nurse, staff nurses work very hard. However, all nurses work either shifts or during the daytime only and so have much shorter working hours than the doctors.

Staff nurses are usually addressed as 'staff' rather than 'nurse' and wear a uniform that distinguishes them from the other grades. This is often a plain dress in a colour other than green, and their hats are marked with a single broad stripe. Male staff nurses are addressed in the same manner and usually wear a white tunic with epaulettes which match the colour of the uniform dresses.

SEN or enrolled nurse (formerly, state enrolled nurse)
This is the second largest group of qualified nurses on the ward. SENs perform many of the roles of the staff nurse but promotion is not possible directly from this grade. This group includes a large number of very experienced nurses, often more highly valued than less experienced staff nurses, despite their lesser qualification. SENs usually wear a plain green uniform in contrast to the staff grade, and have a single broad green stripe on their hat.

Nursing auxiliary
These nurses have no formal qualifications but are given a short training course and are then employed on the ward to perform many of the less skilled tasks. Training continues on the ward and they provide assistance for qualified members of staff. They usually have no direct responsibility for patient care. The uniform is a plain gingham dress, often in brown. Like the SENs this grade often includes the slightly older nurse with a greater experience in life.

Pupil nurses
Student nurses presently do much of the day-to-day work on the ward and sometimes carry considerable responsibility. This is the result of staff shortages on the ward, particularly at night. Often a ward will be run by only a single qualified nurse, accompanied by pupil nurses. Pupil nurses vary widely in their knowledge and skills, from the absolute beginner to the nearly qualified. The time they have spent in training is indicated by the number of thin stripes on their hats (as opposed to the single broad stripe on the hats of qualified nurses). Thus a single green stripe signifies the first year of training of a pupil SEN and three stripes, perhaps blue, signifies the final year of a pupil staff nurse.

Pupil nurses will be intimately involved in your personal care as each will be allocated a certain number of patients. You will probably have the same nurse looking after you on certain shifts throughout your hospital stay and this familiarity will make your stay more comfortable.

The Ward Sister
The sister has overall responsibility for nursing care on her ward and will closely supervise her nursing staff. In addition, the sister has an administrative role including financial responsibility for the ward budget. Some older ward sisters have held posts for many years and can remember the consultants as junior doctors! This gives them an influence that extends well beyond their rank and

even consultants will defer to their greater experience. As a houseman, I was fortunate to have a very experienced sister to guide me through the early days but you can be sure I was careful to cultivate a good relationship! A good sister will take responsibility for many of the minor decisions that would otherwise occupy the overworked houseman.

The very experienced sisters have a sixth sense about patients and their progress. I can remember numerous occasions as a houseman when a developing complication was anticipated by the sister, well in advance of my recognising the problem. The whole atmosphere on a ward depends very much on the sister and the relationship she has with the other nurses on the ward. If you have any difficulty with the staff, or worries about your treatment, sister is a good person to consult. Most sisters join in with the other nurses in direct patient care and will try and get to know all the patients. They are also very skilled at communicating with relatives and will often be able to set minds at rest or sort out misunderstandings.

Sisters are often distinguished by a dark blue uniform or else a frilly white cap or arm bands. The male equivalent of the sister is the charge nurse who has a different title but exactly the same responsibilities. His rank is usually made clear by a name badge.

Theatre department nurses

Another place you will meet nurses is in the operating theatre recovery ward. Following an operation, the anaesthetist will accompany each patient to the recovery ward where an individual nurse will be assigned to supervise the patient's recovery. These nurses are specially trained in the needs and problems of the post-operative patient. They are skilled at looking after semi conscious patients and will make sure that breathing and circulation are satisfactory. They also commonly administer the first dose of pain killer after an operation. Some recovery wards function as post-operative intensive care units and the staff here will be skilled in the care of critically ill patients.

Another large group of nurses you probably won't meet but who will care for you are the operating theatre staff. These nurses have specialised training in surgery and provide vital assistance for the surgeon. They look after all the surgical instruments and other sterile supplies and work closely with the surgeon during each operation. Like the surgeon, they 'scrub' and don sterile gowns, gloves, hats and masks.

OPERATING DEPARTMENT ASSISTANT (ODA)

Almost every patient having an operation will meet an ODA in the anaesthetic room, although in some hospitals, much the same job is performed by anaesthetic nurses. ODAs are highly trained and skilled technicians who provide assistance for the anaesthetist. When you come into the anaesthetic room before your operation, the ODA will check your identity and confirm what operation you are having. He will attach the various monitors to you and will assist the anaesthetist when your anaesthetic begins. Once you are asleep, he will help the anaesthetist transfer you to the operating table and position you carefully so that you come to no harm. Modern anaesthetic practice may involve very complex and sophisticated equipment and the ODAs are responsible for maintaining and helping to operate this equipment. In an emergency, the ODAs are skilled at resuscitation and providing advanced life support. The role of the ODA is so vital that in most hospitals, there is a strict rule that no anaesthetic is started without the presence of an ODA. These important staff deserve much wider recognition than they enjoy at present.

PHYSIOTHERAPISTS

These highly trained and skilled staff play a major role in post-operative recovery. They are not nurses but train for three years before taking the examinations of the Chartered Society of Physiotherapy. You can identify physiotherapists by their navy blue uniform trousers and white tunic.

Physiotherapists use a wide variety of physical therapies to assist in healing, return of physical function and prevention of complications. They are particularly concerned with the skeleton, joints and muscles and the application of exercise to rebuild strength and flexibility. You will come across examples of their work when you read about the post-operative recovery of the four patients later in this book.

Any patient having a major abdominal or chest operation will meet the physiotherapist, often before surgery. You will be taught breathing exercises and will have regular sessions of physiotherapy after your operation to prevent segments of the lung collapsing and causing chest infection. In addition, you will be taught exercise for your legs and abdomen, to keep these moving and prevent other complications such as deep venous thrombosis. These simple therapies are crucially important and in some instances, life saving. For this reason there is always a physiotherapist on call twenty-four hours a day in the hospital.

If you are having an operation on a limb, or on your spine, you will spend a lot of time in the physiotherapy department relearning to use the affected part and overcoming post-operative stiffness and weakness. Patients with major injuries or operations to their legs may have to be taught to walk again.

Physiotherapists work with a very wide variety of patients and now also use a sophisticated range of ultrasound and other devices to lessen pain and speed healing. The full extent of their work is much too wide to describe here and includes the challenge of returning function to patients severely disabled, for instance after a stroke.

OCCUPATIONAL THERAPISTS

Most of us take for granted that we can easily perform day to day tasks like dressing, washing, cooking, opening a can and the many other actions that make up our day. However, if you are injured, disabled, are elderly or infirm, you may not manage all these tasks and your independence will be threatened. Occupational therapists specialise in the study of everyday tasks and find solutions to these problems so that independence may be regained. You will recognise these staff on the ward by their green trousers and white tunics.

Their approach is manifold. A whole variety of simple aids may make life much easier such as hand rails in bathrooms and ramps instead of steps. Ingenious devices make it possible to put on stockings and shoes without bending over. Extensions to tap handles and specially designed can-openers, knives and forks allow the weak hand to function. Alternative techniques of dressing or washing bypass disabilities. The options are endless.

Occupation of the mind with worthwhile pastimes and hobbies and relearning social skills also play a part in rehabilitation from injury or illness. New skills are taught to permit re-employment.

The great majority of patients having operations will not need the occupational therapist. But if you are elderly and live alone, or have any disability, you may spend much of your time in the occupational therapy department once you are mobile after your operation. Initial assessment of individual patients is done on the ward and then you will visit the department, a cheerful and busy place where much social activity goes on. You may be taken through a typical day and asked to perform specific tasks like boiling a pan on the stove. This is the only way in which specific difficulties may come to light. When the time of your discharge from hospital approaches, a home visit may be arranged in which staff from the department take you home to make a detailed report of the difficulties you face, and what aids might be fitted.

RADIOGRAPHERS

These are the technicians who work in the x-ray department and operate x-ray machines and the various types of body scanners. The increasing complexity and sophistication of imaging techniques has meant that these staff now need to be very highly trained. Not only do they understand the workings of the machines but they are also skilled at moving and positioning patients to get the best results. They work closely together with the radiologists.

X-ray departments are very busy places through which pass many hundreds of patients a day. Even with the best of planning, there are inevitable difficulties and delays and sometimes the need to fit in emergency cases. So if you are kept waiting, try to be patient.

In the course of a career, staff in an x-ray department are exposed to many thousands of x-ray doses. Like all other forms of radiation, small doses are harmless but repeated doses may have cumulative damaging effects in the long term. For this reason, radiographers will take every precaution to minimise their own exposure to x-rays and will either wear a lead coat or disappear behind a screen when an x-ray is taken. Do not be alarmed. The very tiny doses of x-rays you receive will not harm you.

PHARMACISTS

To become a pharmacist, you need to take a three- or four-year degree course and then spend a further year in practical training before registration. Hospital pharmacists keep and dispense a huge number of drugs and also closely survey drug prescriptions within the hospital. Doctor's prescriptions are monitored almost daily and possible problems such as cross-reaction between two different drugs are notified to the medical staff. Policy recommendations are made about the use of common drugs like antibiotics and a careful eye is kept on drug cost. Pharmacists provide doctors with detailed advice about particular prescribing problems. Often, specialised services such as intravenous feeding are organised and supplied by the pharmacy department. Pharmacists visit the wards to consult with staff and oversee prescriptions and you will also see them in the hospital dispensary.

DIETICIANS

Many patients in hospital have nutritional problems, through illness, starvation, or inability to take normal food. Wound healing and general recovery depend on good nutrition as I discussed earlier. Surgical patients may have special problems of nutrition particularly if they have a condition or operation affecting the digestive tract. A dietician is trained to understand and treat these problems by the use of specialised or supplemented diets. Problems they deal with range from simple weight loss and protein deficiency to diabetes or the inability to swallow solid food. If you have a nutritional disorder, the dietician will come and talk to you and to the houseman to diagnose the problem. A special individual diet will then be designed and supplied for you and the dietician will keep a careful eye on your progress.

MEDICAL SOCIAL WORKER

Many patients receive state pensions or benefits. Your entitlement to these changes when you are admitted to hospital and this may be a source of confusion and worry. Also, following your operation, you may need the support of social services and, especially if you live alone, there may be many arrangements to deal with. For instance, you may have problems with housing, heating, finances, shopping, provision of meals, or the care of pets. All of these problems are the concern of the medical social worker who can mobilise services such as home help and meals-on-wheels to support your independent existence.

These social workers are based in hospitals but are employed by the DHSS. They can give you detailed advice about benefits and will help you complete the necessary forms. They will act as liaison between the many different agencies involved in your care and if necessary can contact your family or neighbours to arrange help and support. If you are to leave home and move into residential care, the social worker will help with the arrangements. In complex cases, all the hospital staff will meet together to coordinate a plan to get a patient home with the necessary support. Thus the houseman would meet with the ward sister, physiotherapist, occupational therapist, social worker and sometimes a concerned relative.

If you have any worries or problems along these lines, tell any of the staff on the ward and the medical social worker will come and see you. They are specially trained to deal with problems arising out of medical conditions or disabilities and will maintain confidentiality. If they need to discuss your condition with anyone other than the hospital staff or their own professional colleagues, they must first obtain your permission.

DOMESTIC STAFF

There was once a survey to find out who spent most time talking to patients on the hospital ward. Was it the doctors, nurses, porters, or perhaps physiotherapists? No, in fact the domestic staff came first, followed by nurses, with doctors well down the league!

The domestic staff are employed to clean the wards and corridors and serve meals. Traditionally, these are cheerful, talkative people who enormously enjoy their contact with the patients. One sad aspect of modern hospital life is that the quiet broom and mop have been replaced by noisy machines that make conversation impossible. Increasingly, domestic services are being run by private contractors and this further reduces the social aspect of their work.

PORTERS

Without porters, any hospital would seize up almost instantly. No patient is moved anywhere and none of the vital supplies are delivered to any department without a porter. Even the meals for patients have to be delivered by porters. Blood specimens would never reach the laboratories, notes would never leave the records department and drugs would remain locked in the pharmacy were it not for porters. If you have to travel between any two parts of the hospital during your stay, a porter will come and fetch you, most commonly with a wheelchair. When it is time for your operation, a theatre porter will come to the ward with a trolley to collect you.

Most porters, like taxi drivers, are sociable people who like having a chat and enjoy meeting people. They are a fund of intimate information about how the hospital works and will always be happy to answer your questions.

5 Tests

One aspect of coming into hospital that many people fear is the barrage of tests they may be subjected to. This chapter explains why tests need to be done, how they can help your treatment and whether you are likely to have any.

Tests, or investigations as they are often called by doctors, are done for a number of different purposes. Many surgical conditions can be reliably diagnosed by careful attention to the symptoms and the findings on physical examination. If, in addition, the patient is young and fit, there is no point in doing any tests. If an older patient is to have an anaesthetic, then some simple tests ought to be done beforehand because there is a reasonable chance that some abnormality would be found that might affect the anaesthetic. For instance, the older patient might have an electrocardiogram to check the heart rhythm, a chest x-ray, and blood tests to exclude anaemia or reduced kidney function. Doing tests on the off chance that something abnormal might be found is called screening. Screening everyone is a fruitless and costly exercise because the yield of abnormal results is so low. Therefore, screening is applied only to certain groups in which there is a higher chance of detecting significant abnormality.

Many other surgical conditions require investigations to confirm the diagnosis. For instance, the symptoms of gallstones may be mimicked by other common conditions and an ultrasound scan can be used to visualise the gall bladder and demonstrate the presence of stones. Sometimes, a condition that has already been diagnosed needs to be quantified. For instance, the extent of spread of a tumour may be revealed by a body scan. A patient who is having a major operation will need repeated tests after the operation to monitor their progress. These tests will also need to be done before the operation so that a baseline is established with which to compare the subsequent results.

These are some of the different sorts of tests that can be done:

- Blood tests
- Urine tests
- X-rays
- Body scanning
- Endoscopy
- Electrocardiogram

BLOOD TESTS

Hundreds of blood tests are now routinely available in the hospital laboratory. A smaller number of these are performed so commonly that most hospitals now have sophisticated machines that automatically perform the measurements and put the results on computer.

Before I explain about those, a practical word about having the blood sample taken. Many people find themselves bruised after a blood test. This is entirely unnecessary. The bruising is caused by the leak of a small quantity of blood from the vein into the surrounding tissues. The pressure inside veins is very low so this leak is easily prevented by gentle pressure over the puncture site. The hole will very quickly seal itself with a clot. The most common site for taking blood samples is at the elbow crease and there is a long-standing tradition of asking the patient to bend the elbow immediately after the needle is withdrawn. Although this works satisfactorily in some cases, often a bruise will be left behind. The solution is to keep the arm straight and apply gentle pressure for a minute with a finger. This is something you can easily do yourself.

Blood count

This is one of the commonest tests. Blood is composed of red cells that carry oxygen, white cells that fight infection, platelets that are tiny cell fragments important in blood clotting, and a clear fluid called plasma in which all these are bathed. A blood count measures the numbers of these cells and platelets and also gives information about the size and contents of the cells. The substance in the red cells that carries oxygen is called haemoglobin. A deficiency in haemoglobin is called anaemia and this can be caused by a wide variety of conditions or by bleeding. The blood count measures the haemoglobin concentration and if this was very low, then a blood transfusion would be given. In major operations, the blood loss can be considerable so a check blood count will be done after the operation to measure this loss.

The number of white cells in the blood can increase very rapidly in response to infection or inflammation. The white blood cell count is therefore very helpful in trying to diagnose conditions such as acute appendicitis or a chest infection.

The platelet count is rarely abnormal but several conditions do exist in which the number of platelets is dramatically reduced. Surgery, when the platelet count is low, could result in severe bleeding but a transfusion of platelets can be given before an operation, to remedy this deficit.

Some races from tropical parts of the world have a high incidence of inherited blood conditions such as sickle cell anaemia. An acute attack of sickle cell can be triggered by problems during an anaesthetic but precautions can be taken if the condition is recognised. Any patient of Caribbean origin, for example, will have a blood count to screen for this condition before an operation. If anaemia is detected, the specific test for sickle cell would then be done.

Blood chemistry

Plasma contains a very large number of salts, proteins, enzymes and other trace substances that can tell us much about the health of the internal organs. The most common blood tests measure urea and electrolytes, usually abbreviated to U&Es. Urea is a waste product of protein breakdown and is constantly produced by the body. It is excreted in the urine by the kidneys and a rise in urea concentration is a signal that kidney function is impaired. The electrolytes are salts such as sodium and potassium whose concentrations are closely regulated in the plasma. The function of nerves and muscles, including the heart muscle, depend critically on this regulation and a disturbance in the concentration of potassium can lead to serious irregularities of heart rhythm. This risk is heightened by surgery and anaesthesia. Failing kidney function can lead to a dangerous rise in potassium concentrations and some drugs can also disturb the regulating mechanism. Therefore, usually anyone over 50 years old, or anyone taking these sorts of drugs will have their U&Es checked before an anaesthetic.

With increasing age, a mild form of diabetes is very common. This is signalled by an abnormally high level of sugar in the blood before any symptoms emerge. In the older patient it should be routine to check the blood sugar although a simple test for sugar in the urine will detect most diabetics.

The other blood chemistry tests performed most often on surgical patients are called 'liver function tests', or LFTs. In fact these are tests more of liver damage or dysfunction than function but are very helpful in determining the cause of yellow jaundice, for instance. Jaundice is the sign of abnormally high levels of a yellow pigment called bilirubin, normally excreted by the liver into the bile. Damage or inflammation in the liver causes certain enzymes to leak out of liver cells into the blood stream and the levels of these are measured together with bilirubin. In addition, the concentration of important blood proteins, manufactured by the liver, are measured. Serious malnutrition would be reflected in abnormally low concentrations of these plasma proteins.

Cross-matching

Any patient having a major operation may need a blood transfusion, either during or after the operation, to replace blood losses. Blood from another person may be recognised by your own immune system as foreign, resulting in rapid destruction and fragmentation of the transfused blood cells within the circulation. This can have disastrous, even fatal consequences. To find blood that is safe to transfuse, first the right blood group must be chosen, then a number of different donor blood types must be tested to see if they react with your blood. This process is called cross matching and only donor blood that doesn't react will be supplied for transfusion in a particular patient. Mistaken identity could be disastrous so identity is carefully checked, both when the blood sample is taken from you and when the transfusion is given.

URINE TESTS

One of the advances of modern medicine is accurate, cheap and reliable testing of urine on the ward. Thin plastic strips, costing just a few pence, are coated with separate bands of chemical reagents which respond with a change in colour. The strip is simply dipped in urine and within seconds, the abnormal presence of sugar, blood, protein or bilirubin is revealed, even in microscopic traces. This can give early warning of diabetes, kidney disorders, cystitis and jaundice. If abnormal results are found, these can be backed up by more thorough testing in the laboratory. This test is so simple and cheap that almost every patient in hospital ought to have it done at least once. Often the test is routinely performed in the outpatient clinic.

Cystitis, an inflammation of the bladder caused by infection of the urine, is relatively common in hospital patients, especially if they have a urinary catheter (a tube to empty the bladder). This needs to be treated with antibiotics which should be chosen according to the type of infection. Urine culture is the name for the test in which a sample of the urine is incubated together with nutrients to detect the presence of bacteria. The bacteria multiply in number and can then be identified and tested against different antibiotics.

X-RAYS

Everyone knows that x-rays show up the bones of the body. What is not generally appreciated is that many of the soft tissues of the body also cast subtle shadows on an x-ray film and these can give us much information. The best example is the chest x-ray. This shows the bones of the spine, ribs, shoulder blades and the collar bones. But of more interest to the doctor are the shadows cast by the heart and lungs. The shape and size of the heart can be seen. A characteristic outline betrays various different heart conditions. Heart failure leads to accumulation of fluid within the lungs and this can be seen as hazy shadowing. Pneumonia, where parts of the lung become congested with pus, shows a denser shadow. A lung cancer may show as an isolated round shadow.

A plain x-ray of the belly shows faint outlines of the liver and kidneys. A distinctive pattern of gas and fluid levels is seen in obstruction of the bowel. But in general, little can be learnt from plain x-rays of the belly. The solution to this problem is the use of contrast media which cast strong shadows on an x-ray film. This can be used to fill a hollow organ like the stomach or bladder which then shows up in clear outline. A refinement of this technique is to introduce only a little contrast medium and then inflate the organ with air. A very thin film of contrast coats the internal lining of the organ and works just like the dusting powder which betrays fingerprints. The x-rays show every detail of the lining with astonishing clarity. This is the basis of the barium enema.

Barium enemas

Barium is a thick, heavy, white paste which is harmless to tissues but which shows up strongly on an x-ray film. Minutely detailed pictures of the whole large bowel can be obtained if this is used to coat the bowel lining. The lining of the bowel is composed of very active, fast growing tissue and this is where cancers start or where inflammatory conditions of the bowel take place. A barium enema is therefore a very sensitive test for these conditions which show up with a characteristic 'fingerprint'. Having a barium enema can be something of an ordeal so I'll explain what happens.

First of all, the bowel has to be completely emptied. This process starts several days in advance with a diet which produces a low residue in the bowel. This is followed by one or more doses of a very powerful laxative which causes profuse diarrhoea. For an elderly or sick person this can be very debilitating and can cause serious dehydration. You should aim to drink as much as possible to replace fluid losses but stay away from too much tea or coffee as these have a diuretic action which increases fluid loss in the urine. The best type of drink is that sold in chemists, specially for diarrhoea.

When you come to the x-ray department you will be asked to change from your own clothes into a hospital gown. You will be led into an x-ray room which has an electrically powered table with the x-ray machine suspended above. At the touch of a button, the table can be moved in any direction, including a steep tilt to the foot or head end. You will be asked to lie on your side on the table and the small enema tube will be gently inserted into your back passage with the aid of some lubricating gel. This is not painful. About half a pint of barium, as a thick white liquid, will be run into your back passage and this gradually travels up the bowel. When your bowel is completely empty, the sides collapse together. To obtain the detailed x-ray pictures, the bowel must be inflated with air so that the sides come apart and are coated with only a thin film of the barium. The air is introduced through the same small tube by pumping with a rubber bulb like that used for measuring blood pressure. This can be embarrassing as the 'wind' often leaks out with a rude noise. Don't worry. The radiographers are very used to this and at least it's only clean air without any smell. Sometimes the pumping of air can be a little uncomfortable with a colicky discomfort, like natural 'wind'.

Although snapshot x-rays are taken of the various parts of the bowel, most of the information comes from the x-ray pictures which appear on a television screen as the examination is done. Quite often you will be able to watch the pictures yourself and this is a fascinating if rather eerie experience. A radiologist will carefully scrutinise the pictures as the barium flows along the bowel. To reach all the different parts, you will need to be tipped in various directions, by moving the table, so that the barium flows round the corners. This can be very disconcerting especially if the table is tipped very steeply as you may feel rather unsafe. Try and relax. You are in very expert and professional hands. The whole examination takes about half an hour.

The barium is quite harmless to the bowel and will be passed over several days, mixed in with your normal bowel motions, making them a rather pale colour.

IVP (Intra-venous pyelogram)

This is an x-ray of the kidneys and urinary tract, now more properly called an IVU, intravenous urogram. Like a barium enema, this technique uses a contrast medium to enhance the x-ray pictures. When you are positioned on the x-ray machine, the contrast is injected into a needle in a vein on your arm. This mixes with the blood and is rapidly distributed around the whole body in very dilute form. This causes no ill effect apart from an occasional sensation of heat in the skin. The contrast medium has a special affinity for the kidneys which very rapidly extract it from the blood and excrete it in concentrated form in the urine. If a series of x-rays are taken at time intervals, the various phases of excretion show up, first as a blush within the kidney tissues, then as an outline of the urinary tract, down to and including the bladder. An IVP will show up kidney stones, blockages in the draining system and abnormalities of the shape, size and concentrating ability of the kidneys.

Other uses of contrast media

Contrast media can be used in many other ways, to outline parts of the body that don't show on plain x-rays. For instance, narrowing of arteries can be demonstrated by injecting contrast upstream and following its passage with x-ray pictures. Thrombosis in a vein of the leg is shown by injecting into the foot. Compression of spinal nerves by a slipped disc can be pictured by injecting contrast into the spinal fluid that bathes the nerve roots. There are many other examples, too numerous to mention here.

BODYSCANNING

Nowhere has high technology been more successfully applied to medicine than in the development of various kinds of body scanner. These sophisticated machines produce images of the internal organs that were unthinkable only a few years ago. Now almost every district general hospital has a CT (Computer-assisted tomography) scanner and these have already saved many lives by diagnosing blood clots on the brain which require urgent surgery. Tumours or swellings of internal organs can be imaged in fine detail, allowing surgery to be planned, or uncertain diagnoses confirmed.

There are now four types of body scanner, employing different physical principles to produce an image. I will describe each in turn.

Ultrasound scanners

A whole generation of women have experienced ultrasound scanners because they are used in antenatal clinics to check on the condition and growth of babies before they are born.

Instead of x-rays, ultrasound scanners use extremely high frequency sound waves of pitch a hundred times higher than we can hear. These sound waves have a very short wavelength and so are reflected like echoes from even microscopic structures. The principle is exactly the same as sonar, but on a microscopic scale. The scanner detects millions of tiny echoes and uses a computer to work out the position of the structures that reflect the sound waves. These are displayed on a television screen as a cross-sectional picture of the tissue being scanned. Interfaces between solid tissue and liquid show up particularly well, which is why a baby can be seen, floating in the amniotic fluid. Some objects, like gall-stones, cast a sonar 'shadow' and show up very clearly. As far as is known, the sound waves are completely harmless. There is no discomfort for the patient and the machines are small and easily portable. The area of the body to be examined is covered with a special jelly which transmits the sound waves. A small, hand-held probe is then placed against the skin and moved in various directions to obtain the clearest pictures.

A specialised form of ultrasound scanner is used for visualising the heart and this gives moving pictures showing the action of the heart's pumping chambers and valves.

CT scanners

These were the first generation of whole body scanners and were invented and developed in Britain. The scanning machine consists of a large doughnut shaped ring, standing upright. The hole through the middle is big enough to admit an adult lying on a narrow motorized table which moves the subject through the scanner in small steps. At each position, the machinery within the doughnut moves in a complete circle around the subject making thousands of measurements of x-ray absorption at different angles. A very powerful computer then performs complex calculations to deduce the internal structure of the body at that level. This is displayed on a television screen as a cross sectional slice right through the body, showing all the organs in clear detail. The subject is then moved another centimetre into the machine and another scan made. A complete picture of any part of the body can be built up by examining each of the slices in turn, rather like slices in a loaf of bread.

Having a CT scan is a rather eerie experience. The scanning room in the x-ray department will be purpose built and empty apart from the dominating machine. Usually there is a large window set in one wall with a view from the control room. You will be positioned on the table and may be secured with straps as any movement during the scan will blur the picture. If a scan is being made of your chest or abdomen, you will be asked to hold your breath for the duration of each scan, usually about five or ten seconds. Once you are positioned, everyone else will leave the room until all the scans are done. During the scan the machine makes quite a loud whirring noise and if you are required to hold your breath, a recorded voice is sometimes used to make the instructions.

'Breathe in. . . Hold your breath!. . . Relax!'

With the completion of each scan, the table will move you a short distance through the scanner. The scanner room is equipped with a television camera and microphone and also a loudspeaker to allow communication between the patient and the staff in the control room. You will be watched continuously and your voice can be heard in the control room. The reason for your isolation is the same as I mentioned earlier, to protect the staff from repeated x-ray exposure. The small dose you receive from the scanner will do you no harm.

Magnetic resonance imaging (MRI)

This is the latest breakthrough in scanning technology and, so far, few hospitals have been able to afford the price tag of a million pounds or more. These scanners produce images of dramatic clarity and detail and moreover, can synthesize cross-sectional views in several different directions. Thus, a detailed image of the whole length of the spinal cord can be displayed, for instance, rather than the sliced-up images of the CT scanner.

Although the MRI scanner looks rather like a CT scanner, it works on a completely different principle and doesn't expose the subject to any x-rays. To obtain an image, the subject is placed in an extremely powerful magnetic field produced by a super-conducting magnet within the machine. The effect of this is to line up the magnetic poles of individual atoms in the body, rather like compass needles. A very brief burst of radio energy is then transmitted by the scanner, which is tuned to the natural magnetic resonant frequency of hydrogen atoms. The atoms respond by vibrating briefly about their pole position. Because of the way they are all lined up, a coherent 'echo' can be detected by a very sensitive receiver and the returning signals are fed into a computer. Rather like the CT scanner, the computer combines all these signals into a clear image by complex calculation.

So far, no ill effect has been demonstrated from the use of these powerful magnetic fields, unlike x-rays which are definitely damaging after high cumulative doses. The subject experiences no sensation during the scan but care must be taken to remove all metal objects, including jewelry, from the vicinity of the scanner because any metal object would be powerfully attracted by the magnet.

Gamma camera

This is a specialised type of scanner used to image a single organ at a time. A substance is injected that has a high affinity for the particular organ being studied. This substance is labelled with a very weak dose of radioactive atoms which rapidly decay, emitting gamma radiation in the process. Unlike the radioactive elements found in a nuclear reactor which have half lives of thousands of years, the radio-labels used in medical imaging lose all their radioactivity in hours or days and the total dose of radiation is very tiny. The substance is concentrated in the particular organ from which varying densities of gamma radiation are emitted. The gamma camera is positioned over the patient and detects the pattern of gamma rays. A rather coarse and speckled picture is obtained which outlines the organ. Sometimes a computer is used to generate a multicoloured image, with different colours for different densities of gamma rays.

The advantage of this technique is the information it gives about blood flow to the different parts of the organ. For instance, a lung perfusion scan shows the distribution of blood flow to the lungs. If one of the blood vessels in the lung is blocked by a blood clot (pulmonary embolus), this region of the lung shows up as a hole in the image, because the radio-labelled substance can't get to that part of the lung. In contrast, a bone scan may show 'hot spots' where there is increased blood flow indicating inflammation of a joint, for instance.

By using substances which concentrate in various different organs, scans can also be made of the heart, brain, kidneys, liver, spleen and thyroid gland. Typically, a scan takes about half an hour and involves no more discomfort than an intravenous injection and lying still on a table in front of the gamma camera.

ENDOSCOPY

This simply means direct vision of the internal passages of various organs by the use of a telescope inserted through a natural orifice. The stomach, large bowel, bladder and lungs can be examined in this way and the technique has been revolutionized by the introduction of fibre optics. The Japanese led the development of these new telescopes because they have a very high incidence of stomach cancer and wanted to detect these cancers at an early stage by direct vision of the stomach. The fibre optic telescope contains a bundle of thousands of glass fibres, each as fine as a hair, and very flexible. A lens focuses the image on one end of the bundle which then transmits the image, even around corners, to the eye-piece of the telescope. The larger telescopes, about as thick as a finger, are more than a metre in length and can reach around the entire large bowel. The tip can be steered in different directions to explore an organ. The telescope also contains a very bright light source, channels for irrigation and suction, and a channel for instruments to obtain tissue samples or perform other manipulations. The smallest fibre optic telescopes are only a few millimetres in diameter and can explore all the air passages through the nose and deep into the lungs.

Not only are these telescopes used for diagnostic purposes but surgery can be performed through the telescope without making a single cut. For instance, a small kidney stone can sometimes become lodged in the ureter which is the tube joining the kidney to the bladder. This is a serious condition which causes severe pain and can lead to kidney failure. Formerly, the only treatment was quite a major operation to expose the ureter, cut the stone out and then repair the hole. Now, a common procedure is to guide a telescope up through the bladder into the ureter and grasp the stone in a wire basket. This can then be withdrawn with the telescope.

Most endoscopy is performed without an anaesthetic but under powerful sedation and sometimes with local anaesthetic at the route of entry. The most commonly used sedative is a drug called midazolam which combines a short duration of action with very strong amnesic properties. I have never yet met a patient who could remember anything about their endoscopy even though they were clearly awake and co- operative at the time. To examine the stomach, the patient is asked to swallow the telescope as it is gently pushed down. A lozenge, sucked half an hour before endoscopy, anaesthetises the throat and prevents gagging. Although this would be an unpleasant experience for someone without sedation, after the injection of midazolam, the huge majority of patients accept the procedure without any distress. The large bowel is examined by inserting the telescope gently through the back passage, although the bowel must first be emptied and prepared with laxatives and washouts.

76 · Tests

Most endoscopy is performed as an outpatient procedure in a specialised department. You will attend the hospital in either the morning or afternoon and will go home a few hours later, when the sedative drug has worn off. It is not safe to drive a car on the same day because of the residual effects of the sedative drug.

ELECTROCARDIOGRAM (ECG)

This is a very simple and quick bedside test that reveals much about the health of the heart. With every heart beat, a wave of electrical energy sweeps through the heart muscle in a carefully timed and regulated fashion. This originates in the natural pacemaker of the heart which discharges at regular intervals. If electrodes are attached to the skin, a recording can be made of the direction and magnitude of the electrical impulse. Any dysfunction of the heart including abnormal rhythm, strain of the heart muscle, poor blood supply or an actual heart attack will show up as characteristic changes in the voltage waveform.

The first part of the test is done by attaching electrodes to both wrists and ankles. A switching circuit selects different pairs of limbs to 'look' at the heart from different directions. The second part is a more detailed test with five electrode positions on the front of the chest. The whole examination takes about five minutes and a technician or one of the doctors will bring the ECG machine to you. During the test you must try and relax and lie still because movement of any muscle generates electrical interference which will mask the faint heart signals.

During your operation, an ECG monitor will be used to keep an eye on your heart rhythm. This is a simplified form with wires connected to three electrodes on your chest, rather than your limbs.

WHAT TESTS WILL YOU HAVE PERFORMED?

There is no fixed rule for this. Certain tests are done to aid diagnosis of your condition and these might be performed on patients of any age. Otherwise, anyone who is under fifty years of age, who is generally fit and well and who is having a minor operation, need have no tests except a simple urine test. Anyone over fifty, or those who are unwell or on certain medications ought to be screened with some simple tests before an anaesthetic. For instance, George, who is in his sixties and who is having a major bowel operation, had the following tests:

- Blood tests:

Full blood count, which revealed anaemia
Urea and electrolytes to check kidney function
Liver function tests
Blood cross-match, for transfusion
- Ward urine test
- Barium enema, to confirm the diagnosis of bowel tumour
- Chest x-ray
- Ultrasound scan of liver to exclude tumour spread
- Electrocardiogram

Susan is in her thirties and is having a gall-bladder operation. She had only blood tests, to check for anaemia, to test for jaundice or liver inflammation, and baseline urea and electrolytes, for comparison with post-operative results. Her gallstones were earlier confirmed with an ultrasound scan.

6 The Anaesthetic

Many people fear the anaesthetic more than the surgery itself. This fear is due to popular misconception and several myths. It is sometimes based on former unpleasant experiences, often dental extractions under gaseous anaesthesia in the distant past. One myth is that all patients vomit after a general anaesthesia. Another is that anaesthetists are some sort of technician and not a doctor. An impromptu survey of the patients on my ward revealed that less than half the patients knew that anaesthetists were doctors. Another colourful myth is that patients talk while they are anaesthetised and give away all their secrets!

'Anaesthesia' is a Greek word (anaisthesia) meaning 'lack of feeling'. 'Analgesia' which has a related meaning, is also a combination of Greek words 'a', not or without, and 'algos', pain, which put together means a state of insensitivity to painful stimuli. For instance, aspirin is an analgesic. Ether is an anaesthetic (ie makes you insensitive to all stimuli and therefore unconscious) but ether also has analgesic properties.

The modern science of anaesthetics dates back to 1846 when a Boston dentist named William Morton demonstrated successful anaesthesia on a man having a tumour removed from the side of his neck. The anaesthetic agent he used was ether and the audience of prominent medical men at the Massachusetts General Hospital quickly spread the word of this revolutionary new advance in surgery. Within three months, ether was being used in England. An earlier demonstration of the weaker anaesthetic, nitrous oxide, ended in ridicule and uproar while the patient screamed! Nitrous oxide fell out of favour and did not gain popularity until the 1930s when it was used as an analgesic in childbirth. Combined with oxygen in a 50:50 ratio it is still very widely used for this purpose. Nitrous oxide also forms an important component of modern general anaesthesia when combined with other drugs.

A fundamental advance in anaesthetic practice occurred in 1942. Tubocurarine, the active ingredient of a South American arrow poison, was administered to a patient and caused temporary but complete muscular paralysis and relaxation. At first sight, this would seem a dangerous and unhelpful action but in fact it greatly facilitates many operations and paradoxically has made general anaesthesia much safer. Let's find out why. . .

HOW A GENERAL ANAESTHETIC WORKS

An anaesthetist aims to produce three effects in his patient:

1. Sleep (narcosis)
2. Relief of pain (analgesia)
3. Muscle relaxation

'Hang on a sec!' I hear you say, 'Why bother with analgesia when the patient is asleep and can't feel anything? A good point. However, consider this: What happens if you go up to a sleeping man and stick a pin in him? He wakes up with a shout, arms raised, ready to fight, his heart racing, adrenalin flowing. Even though he was asleep, his brain has registered the painful stimulus and has triggered off a whole set of reflex actions with considerable effects on his heart, blood pressure and circulation. The same reflex actions occur when someone is more deeply unconscious under an anaesthetic. So, although the patient doesn't wake up, there are still profound changes within the body in reaction to the surgery. In a fit, young patient, these changes probably wouldn't matter but in someone with a weak heart or narrowed blood vessels in the brain, these effects could be very dangerous.

So, in general, the anaesthetist will try to abolish the reaction to all painful stimuli by causing a state of analgesia. In old fashioned anaesthetics, this was achieved by inducing a state of very deep unconsciousness. Not only was this hazardous in itself, but it took a long time to reach this state, it required very large doses of anaesthetic agents and the recovery of consciousness was slow. In modern anaesthetic practice, only a light level of unconsciousness is induced and painful stimuli are blocked using an analgesic drug. This might take the form of a powerful pain-killer like morphine or one of its derivatives, administered by injection. Alternatively, nitrous oxide can be inhaled as part of the anaesthetic gases, as it is an excellent analgesic. Commonly, a combination of the two is used.

In the ideal anaesthetic, the patient will wake up almost immediately after the operation so the anaesthetist needs to ensure that the patient is pain free. This is another good reason to separate out the two components, anaesthesia and analgesia.

'OK' you say, 'I think I understand all that business about putting people to sleep and about stopping pain but what about this muscle paralysis? I don't think I fancy a shot of arrow poison. How will I be able to breathe if I'm paralysed?'

Muscle relaxation

Surgeons began to have trouble when operating on the abdomen. Whenever they made a cut in the abdominal wall to reach the insides, a perplexing difficulty arose. At first the abdominal wall muscles would part and good access could be obtained by stretching the straight cut into a diamond shaped opening. Instruments called retractors were employed to hold the cut open.

But as the operation proceeded, the muscles would become more and more tense and the opening through which the surgery had to be done became smaller and smaller! Even worse was trying to sew up the cut at the end of the operation. Because the muscles became so tense, the abdominal contents began to bulge out of the cut and closing the abdomen became very difficult.

In fact, this reaction of the abdominal wall muscles should come as no surprise. For every doctor has recognised this reaction when diagnosing an acute surgical emergency such as appendicitis. One of the cardinal signs of acute appendicitis is rigidity of the abdominal wall on the right side, overlying the appendix. The harder you press on this point, the more tense the muscles become until they assume a board-like rigidity. This phenomenon is called 'guarding' and it is a protective reflex to shield an injured or inflamed organ within the abdomen.

It is this same reaction that may occur during surgery on the abdomen. Cutting or handling either the bowel or the lining membrane of the abdominal cavity causes protective muscle spasm. Before the discovery of drugs that could safely relax muscles, the only option was to give large doses of anaesthetic gases and drugs, thereby inducing very deep unconsciousness. To achieve full muscle relaxation, a depth of anaesthesia approaching coma and death was required. Not only was this hazardous but it took a long time for the patient to recover from this deep anaesthesia.

So the demonstration of curare, a drug that caused temporary muscle paralysis and relaxation, revolutionized anaesthesia. The concept of 'balanced anaesthesia' was born. Instead of using a single anaesthetic agent such as ether to produce anaesthesia, analgesia and muscle relaxation in a deeply unconscious patient, a combination of drugs could be used to produce these desired effects in a patient only lightly unconscious. The beauty of this system is that each anaesthetic can be carefully tailored to the requirements of the individual patient and operation. There is now a wide choice of analgesics, anaesthetics and muscle relaxants, each with slightly differing properties and side effects, and part of the skill of the anaesthetist is in choosing the best combination. Further refinement is added by the use of drugs that have a reverse action, for example, counteracting the action of muscle relaxants to restore full muscle power within minutes of injection.

One of the consequences of complete muscle paralysis is that the victim is unable to breathe. This is how the deadly South American arrow poison works, causing death from asphyxia. Clearly, this is not desirable in hospital patients! The anaesthetist must therefore take over the work of breathing of the patient. In medium or longer operations, a tube is placed in the patient's windpipe and connected to a breathing machine called a ventilator. This arrangement has one very important advantage which is protection of the air passages against inhalation of vomit or secretions. Normally, our air passages are kept clear by several reflexes, the most important of which is the cough reflex. If we accidentally swallow food 'the wrong way' and it begins to go down the air passage, immediate coughing occurs as a reflex action to expel the food. This is literally a life preserving reflex and in its absence, inhaled matter can block the air passages causing death in minutes, or else cause inhalational pneumonia. As consciousness diminishes, so the reflex becomes weaker. Tragically, many deaths are caused in this way when people vomit after overdoses of drugs or alcohol.

This is a hazard in anaesthetics and is the reason why patients are always starved for at least four hours before a general anaesthetic, to ensure that the stomach is empty and vomiting cannot occur. But with a tube in the windpipe, sealed with an inflatable collar, the airway is completely protected against such mishaps. This is also very important in any operation on the nose, mouth or throat, such as tonsillectomy, because blood may pool in the throat.

So, with this technique, muscle relaxants serve several purposes. After the patient is put to sleep, a rapidly acting muscle relaxant is given by injection. This relaxes all the muscles in the body including those of the face, neck and throat. This creates the ideal conditions for the anaesthetist to visualise the windpipe at the back of the throat and insert the tube. He now has complete control of the patient's airway and breathing. Because all the chest muscles and the diaphragm are also relaxed, he can easily carry out the artificial breathing, either by hand or by machine. And as mentioned before, the ideal conditions of relaxation are produced in the abdomen as well.

This technique has such huge advantages in terms of control and safety that it is commonly used even when muscle relaxation in the abdomen is not required. This and many other advances in anaesthetic practice have made possible much of modern surgery. Dramatic advances such as open heart surgery and surgery on major blood vessels have followed the development of new techniques in anaesthesia. Many of the same techniques and principles have been applied to intensive care, leading to the survival and recovery of critically ill or seriously injured patients. No longer is old age or ill health a bar to surgery and patients 80 or 90 years old have hip replacements and cataract extractions.

WILL I DIE HAVING MY OPERATION?

Just how safe is having an operation? One of the most comprehensive studies of this question was carried out by the Association of Anaesthetists of GB and Ireland in 1980. They collected data on all the operations carried out in about one third of all the hospitals in England, Scotland and Wales. In these hospitals, more than a million operations were carried out in the twelve months of the study, beginning in March 1979. All the deaths that occurred during the anaesthetic or within six days of the operation were recorded. In as many cases as possible, confidential inquiries into the circumstances and causes of death were sought. About half the operations were done as an emergency on a sick or injured patient. Half were routine operations. The average chance of dying was 1 in 280 but remember that this includes all the emergency operations and more than half the deaths were in patients aged seventy or over. Most deaths were due to natural progression of the patient's illness where surgery had been performed as an only chance of survival. It was estimated that the chances of dying solely of the anaesthetic was 1 in 10,000. The purpose of carrying out this study was to discover if any of the deaths were avoidable and what changes should be made to medical practice and training. In other words, this is an attempt to learn from mistakes in those cases where a death might have been avoidable. These lessons have already been applied to the practice of anaesthesia and surgery.

The data for a follow-up study have been collected and the results were published in 1988. This Confidential Enquiry into Peri-Operative Deaths (CEPOD) closely examined the circumstances of all such deaths in three health regions for a twelve month period. Each case was scrutinised by independent experts both in surgery and anaesthesia to discover if there were avoidable factors that contributed to the patient's death. The inclusion of surgical experts in the study allowed a more balanced appraisal of risk, as some deaths previously attributed to anaesthesia were then found to be associated with deficiencies in surgical practice. A revised estimate of the risk of an anaesthetic was made and in nearly half a million operations, only three deaths could be solely attributed to the anaesthetic.

This brings us back to considering the balance of risk and benefit. George has cancer of the bowel. If this is not treated it is almost certain that he will die of the spreading cancer in a year or less. If he also had lung or heart disease, provided that this did not greatly shorten his life expectancy, it would be worth the risk of an anaesthetic and operation to treat the cancer. The increased risk of the anaesthetic would be justified because of the hope of cure of a fatal condition. Fortunately, George is generally very fit and I expect he will come through the operation very well.

John, on the other hand, is not a fit man. He has serious chest disease and a general anaesthetic would pose a much higher risk. In the opinion of his surgeon, the discomfort and disability he suffers as a result of his hernia doesn't justify that risk. He is unlikely to die of his hernia but he might come to harm if given a general anaesthetic. For patients like John, an alternative approach to anaesthesia must be made. A discussion of these alternative types of anaesthetic follows later.

But first, I sense you are worried by something which I mentioned earlier on.

AWARENESS DURING ANAESTHESIA

'Yes, you were explaining the advantage of balanced anaesthesia and you said that the patient is only lightly unconscious. I've read in the papers about people waking up in the middle of their operation, paralysed and unable to move or speak. That sounds terrifying! How do I know that I won't wake up?'

First of all, let me tell you that this is a very rare occurrence. Three million operations are performed each year in the UK and yet only a handful of patients report the horrifying experiences which are described in the press. A much greater number of patients believe they have been aware during some part of the operation but rarely has this been a distressing experience. Most cases arise from the confusion during emergence from the anaesthetic, after the operation, when consciousness may wax and wane. Awareness during some stage of the operation may occur as often as 1 in 500 but this is almost always momentary and because patients are given analgesics as part of the anaesthetic, this is rarely painful or distressing.

The circumstance in which genuine awareness is most likely to occur is during emergency caesarean section. The caesarean is usually done because the undelivered baby is 'distressed' and may die unless delivered very speedily. This situation creates a dilemma for the anaesthetist because in reality he is anaesthetising two patients, both the mother and baby. If the baby is anaesthetised when delivered through the incision in the abdomen, it won't start breathing. This is the most critical time in a new life, when a pair of lungs takes their first breath. Unless the baby has begun to breathe, it won't receive any oxygen and will quickly die. In fact, this risk is now greatly diminished because a specialist baby doctor will be present at every caesarean section and he can support the baby's breathing, with a ventilator if necessary.

To minimise harmful effects on the newborn baby, the anaesthetist aims to keep the mother only lightly unconscious and just occasionally a mother reports a brief period of awareness but very rarely pain. For non urgent caesarean sections, an increasingly popular option is to keep the mother awake deliberately and to perform the operation under epidural anaesthesia. How this works is explained in the section on local anaesthesia.

In all other operations, unplanned awareness is very rare. The same considerations do not apply and the patient can be taken to a deeper level of unconsciousness. Throughout the operation, the anaesthetist will continually monitor and watch the patient. Repeat doses of various drugs such as analgesics may be required during the operation and various signs that these are beginning to wear off will be present. Thus, an increase in pulse rate or blood pressure, or sweating, or tears may indicate that a patient is becoming 'lighter' and more anaesthetic would be administered, or more analgesic given. The anaesthetist will be able to anticipate which parts of the operation cause the strongest stimulation or 'pain' and will deepen the anaesthetic for this period.

The experience of an anaesthetic is dramatised in chapter eight, 'The day of operation'.

LOCAL ANAESTHETICS

The alternative to general anaesthesia, in which the patient is unconscious, is some form of local anaesthetic in which only part of the body is affected. These techniques use local anaesthetic drugs which can be injected in various different ways to produce numbness. The simplest method is injection at the site of operation, as you may have experienced at the dentist, but local anaesthetics are also used in more sophisticated techniques such as epidural anaesthesia. Local anaesthetics have no effect on the patient's level of consciousness and the patient is usually awake. However, they are sometimes used to supplement general anaesthesia and can also be used to provide post-operative pain relief.

The first demonstration of local anaesthesia was in 1884 when a Viennese doctor, Karl Kohler, showed that cocaine could anaesthetise the surface of the eye. Although cocaine is still occasionally used, a variety of other local anaesthetics without such interesting side effects are now employed. The most commonly used local anaesthetic is lignocaine.

All the local anaesthetics work in the same way by blocking the conduction of electrical signals along nerve fibres. To understand how local anaesthetics are used we need to know a little about the anatomy of the nervous system. When we feel the prick of a needle in an arm we would say that the pain is in the arm. This is an illusion, as pain and all the other sensations like touch and temperature exist only in the brain and are projected by the mind to that part of the body where the nerve signals originate. The truth of this surprising statement is illustrated by the condition called sciatica, often caused by a slipped disc. In this condition, the slipped disc irritates nerve roots coming out of the spinal cord, which results in false messages being sent up the spine. The brain interprets these as pain and the mind projects the pain to the buttock and the back of the leg because this is the area served by these nerve roots. The patient feels pain in the leg, no less real, but clearly the pain doesn't exist in the leg.

The whole surface of the body, and to a lesser extent the internal organs, are covered with millions of tiny sensors which can detect injury, heat, cold, touch, pressure and so on. These are individually wired into nerve circuits that travel back to the brain through the spinal cord. Messages to muscles from the brain follow parallel paths in the opposite direction, also through the spinal cord and nerve roots. The consequence of this wiring arrangement is that nerve signals can be blocked with local anaesthetic drugs at many different points on the path between the sensors and the brain, with exactly the same result. Thus to make a hand numb, local anaesthetic could be injected directly into the hand, around the nerve higher in the arm, or around the spinal cord. In all cases, the result would be the same, anaesthesia of the hand, because the brain would receive no signals from that part of the body.

When local anaesthetic is injected, it is gradually absorbed by surrounding blood vessels until the anaesthetic effect wears off. This is important because the 'local' can have the alarming side effect of paralysing muscles, a simple and harmless consequence of the parallel courses of sensory and muscle nerves. Both are blocked simultaneously and a muscle cannot move without command signals from the brain or spinal cord. As the anaesthetic wears off, so full power will return to the muscles. In general, muscle nerves are less susceptible to local and so a weak concentration of the drug can produce numbness without affecting muscle power very much.

I will conclude this chapter with a brief description of the various ways local anaesthetic is used in practice.

LOCAL ANAESTHETIC TECHNIQUES

Local infiltration

This is the simplest method of producing local anaesthesia. Using a fine needle, the anaesthetic solution, for instance lignocaine, is injected into the tissues at the site of operation. Within seconds, the skin will begin to go numb and within a minute it will be completely insensitive. The sensation is like injections at the dentist which numb the gums and teeth.

A refinement of this procedure is used to anaesthetise a toe or finger. Nerves pass up each side of a finger or toe and if local anaesthetic is injected all around the circumference of the digit, all the nerves will be blocked. This 'ring block' anaesthetises the whole finger or toe beyond this point.

Nerve blocks

If the precise anatomy of the nerve supply to the site of operation is known, then the individual nerves can be blocked without having to inject local anaesthetic right at the site of operation. A good example of this is the type of block that John will have for his hernia repair. The skin and tissues just above the groin on each side are supplied by two nerves that run very close together. They emerge from under the crest of your pelvic bone below the waist. They run down in a diagonal direction towards the groins and supply

86 · The Anaesthetic

sensation to almost all the area where an inguinal hernia appears. If a needle is inserted to just the right level next to the pelvic bone, then local can be injected into the tissues surrounding the nerves. Within a few minutes, the inguinal area will go numb. In fact, for John's operation, a third nerve that rises from the bottom of the inguinal area will also have to be blocked.

You may be worrying that all this poking around with needles will itself be painful. You need have no fear. Local acts so rapidly around the tip of the needle that, if a little care is taken, the tissues immediately ahead of the needle tip will be numb before the needle travels any further. My own practice, shared with many, is to start injecting with the very finest needle available and to progress to bigger needles if I need to go deeper.

Nerve plexus blocks

This is an extension of simple nerve blocks. In certain parts of the body, notably the arm, all the nerves that supply that region come together, intertwine, join and branch. This arrangement is called a plexus from the Latin word meaning plaited. The nerves that supply the arm are all derived from the brachial plexus which in its complexity is a favourite subject for examiners of medical students! This lies under the protection of the collar bone but the tail end extends over the roof of the armpit. If local is injected into the roof of the armpit in precisely the right spot, then the whole bundle of nerves can be blocked and the arm will be anaesthetised.

Intravenous local anaesthetic

This is an alternative way to produce anaesthesia of an arm which works by a simple but ingenious principle. The procedure is as follows: Firstly, a needle is placed in a vein on the limb to be anaesthetised. Next, an inflatable tourniquet is wrapped around the upper arm but left loose. The limb is then elevated for three minutes to drain as much blood as possible. The arm may be stroked or a rubber bandage wrapped around to squeeze out even more blood. The pneumatic tourniquet is then inflated so that it grips the upper limb firmly enough to prevent blood flow. This is perfectly safe for a limited period of time. The empty veins of the limb are then filled with local by injecting into the needle. Because the veins form a fine network throughout the tissues, the local is very rapidly distributed and within minutes, the whole limb below the level of the tourniquet becomes completely anaesthetic.

When the operation is completed, the tourniquet is released and the local is gradually removed by the restored blood flow. Sensation will return. This method of anaesthesia was invented by a German surgeon, August Bier, at the turn of the century. Bier's block is often used when fractures of the wrist bones are being set.

EPIDURAL ANAESTHESIA

Epidural and spinal anaesthetics have had a 'bad press' and are feared by many. 'Epidurals' are most commonly used to provide pain relief in childbirth and this is an emotive subject where many issues other than analgesia cloud the issue. In the early popular days of epidural anaesthesia, there were a small number of tragedies where permanent and serious damage was done to the spinal nerves, causing paralysis of the legs. The lesson of these early accidents has been learnt and epidural and spinal anaesthesia is now very safe. Let's consider how an epidural anaesthetic works and some of the things that went wrong in the early days.

Nerves from different parts of the body converge on the spinal cord at multiple levels up and down the spine. An epidural anaesthetic blocks these spinal nerves, equally on the two sides, for a certain distance up and down the spinal cord. Local anaesthetic is injected into the epidural space which surrounds the spinal cord at a slight distance. The spinal cord itself is bathed in a clear fluid which is separated from the epidural space by a tough membrane, the dura. All the spinal nerves pass through the epidural space and this is the site of action of the local anaesthetic.

The local does not run freely within the epidural space and the amount of spread can be varied by injecting different volumes or positioning the patient. The effect is to produce a band of anaesthesia around the body with normal sensation above and below this level.

How is the epidural injection made? Isn't it dangerous poking needles around the spinal cord? Yes, there is a potential danger but just as the surgeon would never contemplate operating without knowing the anatomy of a region, the anaesthetist will use his knowledge of the anatomy of the spine. The needle is inserted carefully between two bones, passing through various ligaments until the epidural space is reached. Each of the ligaments gives a characteristic resistance to passage of the needle so the anaesthetist will know what depth he has reached. When the epidural space is reached, there is a loss of resistance to injection and this is the guide to accurate placement. A syringe with a few ml of air is connected to the other end of the needle. As the ligaments are traversed, there is a very high resistance to injection and if the plunger of the needle is depressed, it bounces back again. When the tip of the needle reaches the epidural space, air is injected very easily, and there is no bounce of the plunger.

With the needle firmly in place, the syringe is disconnected and a very fine plastic tube (about a millimetre in diameter) is passed through the bore of the needle. The angled tip of the needle directs the tube along the epidural space where it is advanced several centimetres beyond the needle. With the tube remaining in place, the needle is pulled out, passing over the length of the tube. The free end of the tube is connected to a filter and all injections to the tube must pass through this filter. The filter has pores so fine that even bacteria cannot pass, a precaution against infection. The skin puncture site is sprayed with antiseptic and the tube is taped to the back with the injection port in a convenient place, commonly over the shoulder.

So far, this procedure will have produced no anaesthetic effect. But if local is injected through the fine tube into the epidural space, a block of several spinal nerves is produced within minutes. This causes anaesthesia of the area they supply. A small test dose is given first, and then the full anaesthetic dose. The beauty of this system is that repeated doses can be given and the tube left in place for several days. This is a superb way of completely abolishing all the pain after certain kinds of operation.

Are there any side effects? One almost invariable effect is a lowering of the blood pressure. For this reason, an epidural anaesthetic is never performed unless the patient has a running drip connected to a vein. The drip will increase the volume of the circulation and compensate for this effect. If an epidural anaesthetic is done low in the spine, nerves to the pelvis and bladder may be effected. In childbirth, this may slightly prolong the labour because the mother cannot push so effectively. There may also be temporary difficulty in passing urine. Finally, if a very intense blockade is produced by larger doses of concentrated local, it is possible to block muscle nerves. This will produce a feeling of weakness, inco-ordination or even complete paralysis of the legs. Don't worry, this is perfectly safe and after a while the sensation and muscular power will return.

So what went wrong in the early days to produce permanent paralysis in a few unfortunate patients? Some accidents were caused by the way that ampoules of local were stored in alcohol baths. A few ampoules had tiny cracks that allowed alcohol to leak into the ampoule, replacing the local. Alcohol instead of local was unwittingly injected, causing permanent damage to the spinal nerves. Ampoules are now stored dry in sterile packaging to avoid this hazard.

Epidural anaesthetics are now very safe. They are used in a variety of ways, as a sole anaesthetic technique, to supplement general anaesthesia, or to provide superb post-operative pain relief. One of the characters in this book, Susan, has an epidural to provide pain relief after her gall-bladder operation.

SPINAL ANAESTHETICS

These work on the same principle as epidurals but are a one-shot technique with only a single injection. A much finer needle is used and this is passed slightly further until it penetrates the membrane surrounding the spinal fluid. Correct placement is shown by a drop of the spinal fluid flowing from the end of the needle. A single small dose of local is then injected through the needle, and the needle removed. This technique is reserved for lower parts of the spine, below the end of the spinal cord, where only spinal nerve roots float free within the fluid. It produces very good anaesthesia of the lower abdomen, the saddle area between the legs, and of the legs themselves. This lasts for some hours.

In contrast to epidurals, it is possible to produce anaesthesia on one side only, by using local which is denser than spinal fluid. This will sink within the spinal fluid and if the patient is on his or her side, very little block will be produced in the uppermost side. Even more than epidurals, a fall in blood pressure is expected and an intravenous drip must be set up. A more intense blockade of nerves to muscles is usual and the patient will often notice marked weakness and inco-ordination of the legs until the 'spinal' wears off.

The commonest operations performed under spinal anaesthetic are emergency repairs of broken hips in elderly women, and 're-boring' of the enlarged prostate gland in elderly men. This avoids the increased dangers of general anaesthetic in elderly and unfit patients.

THE POPPY, MORPHINE, AND ACUPUNCTURE (for the curious)

Morphine is a drug of antiquity, being the active ingredient of opium. Opium is obtained by incising the seed heads of the opium poppy, and collecting the juice that oozes and dries on the surface of the poppy. Heroin (diamorphine) is converted from morphine by a simple chemical process and after ingestion is converted back to morphine in the body. These drugs, and a number of closely related synthetic versions, are the most powerful pain-killers known. In recent years, researchers have found out how these drugs work in the human body. Some pretty astonishing discoveries were made along the way.

To understand the importance of these discoveries, I need to explain about a molecular structure called a receptor, a universal device employed by cells in the body to receive and decode signals. Receptors lie in the surface membranes of cells throughout the body and receive the signals transmitted by nerves and hormones.

Essentially, information is transmitted around the body in two ways: by free hormones that circulate around the blood and influence many organs, and by individual nerve circuits that transmit their information from one specific site to another. To make an analogy, hormones are rather like the Base Lending Rate is to the 'city'. The level of interest changes from time to time, is broadcast widely, and influences the general level of excitement of the financial marketplace. The hormone, insulin, is secreted in response to a meal and conveys a message which can be broadly translated as: 'Right Oh! All you chaps out there in the body's chemical factories. There's a big new load of raw material arrived and I want you to step up production right away!' In contrast, nerve signals are much more like conversations on a telephone line, between two people only.

The question is, when there are many different hormones circulating around the blood, how does the individual cell recognise and act on the presence of insulin alone? The answer lies in the use of receptors, which act as a sort of ignition switch, operated only by the right key. This is quite a good analogy because receptors are large protein molecules with a hollow on the surface corresponding to a key hole. Only a hormone or transmitter molecule of precisely the right shape will fit into the hollow and activate the receptor. In the same way that turning the key in an ignition switch starts a car engine, a hormone molecule locking into the receptor activates a molecular switch to turn on the engines of cellular metabolism. The analogy goes further because if you put the ignition key from Fred Blogg's Ford Escort into your Escort, the key fits in the switch but won't start the engine. In the same way, there are drugs or chemicals that mimic the shape of a hormone molecule and will fit in the receptor without activating it. These can block the action of the hormone by filling up all the receptor sites. Some drugs fit only loosely in the receptor and weakly activate the switch.

Signals are transmitted from nerve to nerve and from nerve to muscle by the same mechanism. An electrical impulse releases a burst of transmitter chemical from the terminal of the nerve. This diffuses across a tiny gap and activates receptors on the other side. A substance that can block a receptor and prevents the action of the hormone or transmitter chemical is called an antagonist.

So what has all this to do with morphine? Well, the scientists trying to find out how morphine works discovered that certain cells in the nervous system had receptors for morphine! Remember, morphine is a chemical derived from a plant. Why were there receptors for a plant chemical in the human brain?! They studied other related pain-killers and found that they also fitted in the same receptors. Weak pain-killers fitted loosely, strong pain-killers fitted closely. By this time, some extraordinary conclusions were being drawn. These cells must be involved in the perception of pain and there was only one possible explanation for the presence of these receptors: the brain must be manufacturing its own natural pain-killers!

News of this exciting discovery shot around the world and stimulated huge research efforts to find and characterise these natural pain-killers, now known as the family of endorphins. The perfect antagonist to morphine and the other opiate drugs was discovered and this drug, called naloxone, can immediately reverse their action without any other side effects, so specific is the receptor mechanism. Naloxone has saved countless lives because it can reverse even an overdose of morphine or heroin. It is a miraculous sight to administer an injection to a drug addict who is minutes from death, deeply unconscious, scarcely breathing and with pin-point pupils, a cardinal sign of opiate drugs. Within a minute they can be fully conscious and delivered from danger. With a slight overdose of morphine, producing potentially dangerous respiratory depression, it is possible to administer a small dose of naloxone which overcomes the breathing problems without abolishing analgesia.

The discovery of endorphins provides a fascinating link between eastern and western medicine. Guess what happens to the level of endorphins in the brain when acupuncture is performed? That's right, acupuncture stimulates the production of the body's own natural pain-killers and this has been scientifically verified. This fascinating discovery has converted many a sceptic and there are now increasing numbers of conventional doctors willing to use acupuncture.

Finally, let me describe a recent scientific experiment about the power of the mind over pain. The researchers studied the pain of dental extraction, for which a large number of volunteers were given pain-killers. Half the volunteers were given dummy pain-killing tablets, identical in appearance to the real ones, and no-one present (not even the researchers) knew which were the real tablets. The individual boxes of tablets were numbered and the allocation of real or dummy tablets was made by a computer using random numbers. Only the computer knew which patients had which tablets. The patients were asked to record how much pain they had before and after the pain-killers.

In the next stage of the experiment, the patients were given tablets of naloxone to reverse the action of the pain-killer and bring the pain back. Only, so crafty were the researchers, that half had real naloxone and half had identical dummy tablets. Again, this was done in a randomized manner and only the computer knew which patients had real naloxone. The patients were not told the expected action of naloxone and were simply asked to record how much pain they had after the second tablet.

Only when the whole experiment was finished and all the results recorded was the code broken and the computer asked to identify what tablets each patient received. The patients fell into four groups.

In the first group, they were given real pain-killers and then real naloxone. Not surprisingly, they recorded good pain relief from the first tablet and many of them said the pain became worse after they took the second tablet.

The second group were given real pain-killers but dummy naloxone. On average, they had good pain relief from the first tablet and a mixture of reactions to the second. Some reported no change, a few that the pain became worse, and some that the pain was lessened. No surprises here.

The third group were given dummy pain-killers and dummy naloxone tablets. In other words, they had no active medicines at all. Now, here was a surprise because a substantial proportion of these patients reported good pain relief! Some said that the pain was completely abolished. This is a demonstration of the placebo effect, well known to doctors, in which powerful suggestion can improve a patient's symptoms and even cure disease. It is a reflection of the profound influence that the mind has over the body.

But the results in the fourth group were the most fascinating. They were given dummy pain-killers and many reported good pain relief, the placebo effect at work. These patients were then given real naloxone, without being told what its action is, remember. Many of the patients who had achieved analgesia by the placebo effect complained that the pain came back when they were given the second tablet, the naloxone! In other words, the placebo analgesic effect must have been mediated by a rise in levels of endorphins, the body's own natural pain-killers. In the same way that naloxone blocks the effect of morphine, it antagonises the effect of endorphins at the same receptors.

This experiment convincingly demonstrated that suggestion, an influence on the mind, could bring about a chemical change in the nervous system that altered the perception of pain. Pain has a psychology all of its own. How much pain you suffer with your coming operation will depend in part on the state of your mind. If you are anxious and constantly fearful of what unknown insults to your body lie ahead, you will suffer more pain than if you are relaxed and informed. The mind has a powerful influence on many other body functions and a positive attitude to your operation may profoundly influence the healing and recovery process.

7 Consent to Operation

What is consent and why is it necessary?

Every day, doctors perform acts that outside medical practice would constitute an assault upon a patient. For instance, a routine physical examination includes deeds that would comprise indecent assault in any other circumstance. The difference between the flesh wound of the mugger's razor and that of the surgeon's scalpel may only be one of intent. What distinguishes these circumstances is the special relationship between patient and doctor and the consent of the patient to these acts.

The relationship between a patient and doctor is governed by a set of rules to deal with these extraordinary circumstances. By law, the doctor owes a duty of care to the patient. This includes attaining a professional standard of skill and expertise, acting in the best interests of the patient and maintaining confidentiality. Under these conditions the patient then gives their consent to the various acts, mentioned before, in the belief that they are performed for the patient's own good. Essentially, the relationship is based on trust, and breaches of that trust by the doctor are termed professional misconduct. Serious professional misconduct may result in a doctor losing his licence to practise and his name is then 'struck off' the Medical Register. Registration of doctors and matters of professional misconduct are dealt with by the General Medical Council.

Without your consent, a doctor is not permitted to examine you, obtain a blood or urine sample, or perform an operation. Often, consent is implied and if you voluntarily attend a doctor's appointment then he will expect you to comply with a request for examination without further discussing the matter. Likewise, if he takes a blood sample without your protest or refusal, he will assume your consent. However, the use to which such a blood sample is put has recently become the subject of much controversy and this will serve to illustrate some of the principles of consent.

The controversy arose with the emergence of the AIDS (Acquired Immune Deficiency Syndrome) epidemic. Many doctors believe that an essential weapon in the fight against the spread of this terrible disease is an accurate knowledge of the distribution of the virus in the population. They advocate doing the blood test for the AIDS virus on a very large sample of the population. One feasible approach would be to perform the AIDS test on every blood sample which is obtained for other routine blood tests. Millions of patients could be tested in this way with little extra cost. But is it ethical? Unless the patient has given their specific consent to the AIDS test, use of any portion of their blood sample in this way would amount to an assault on the patient, even though the patient willingly gave a sample for other purposes.

In principle, this applies to any blood test. In practice, ten or twenty tests are often performed on a single blood sample with only the patient's general consent, because in general routine blood tests have routine results without any profound implications for the patient. On the other hand, the results of the AIDS test, and the knowledge of those results have the most profound implications for the patient. A general principle thus emerges that the degree of consent given by a patient should depend on the implications for the patient of the procedure or investigation. Routine examination and blood tests require only the general (often implied) consent of the patient. Any procedure, such as an operation, with greater implications should only be performed with the patient's explicit consent. The doctor has a duty to inform the patient of the effects and possible hazards of an operation. These may have greatly differing implications for patients depending on their life-styles and personal values. Whether or not an operation is in the interests of a patient is therefore a decision that can often only be made by the patient and not by the doctor. This is the very important principle of informed consent.

This principle has only been recognised in very recent years as a result of changing attitudes towards the medical profession. Until recently, doctors held an authoritarian position and patients accepted whatever treatment was meted out to them because 'doctor knows best'. With the rise of consumerism, that authoritarian stance has been eroded and patient's rights have come to the fore. Just how recent a change this has been is illustrated by a debate on the subject of informed consent, by the Law Lords in 1985. This debate arose out of the final appeal to the House of Lords of an elderly lady suing a surgeon for an operation that had gone wrong.

The late, distinguished neurosurgeon had operated on her spine in an attempt to relieve pressure on nerves causing chronic pain in her arms. A recognised, though rare, complication of this operation is damage to the nerve roots or spinal cord. Unfortunately, the woman suffered this complication and as a result was partially paralysed and permanently disabled. Although she did not criticise the surgeon in his standard of diagnosis or operative skills, she maintained that had she been informed of the risk of this complication, she would not have consented to the operation.

Although her appeal was dismissed by the Lords on the facts of the case, the general issue of informed consent was debated at some length by the Law Lords. Lord Scarman gave a formal legal opinion on the subject which, although not legally binding, is likely to influence the judgement on any future cases.

His judgement was in two parts. Firstly he quoted the Bolam principle which defines the standard of care required of a doctor. This principle is employed in any case where negligence is claimed. If the doctor has acted in accordance with a practice accepted as proper, by a responsible body of medical opinion, he can not be found negligent, even though other doctors adopted a different practice. Furthermore, the acceptability of that practice must be judged by the standards of that time even though practice may have changed since. In other words, although the doctor's duty of care is upheld by the law, the standard of that care is a matter of medical opinion. This was reiterating a well established legal principle.

In the second part of his judgement he broke new ground. When the lady had her operation, many years before, it was not the standard practice to inform patients of possible complications. A responsible body of medical opinion would therefore judge that the surgeon's practice in omitting to warn of complications was proper. He could not, therefore, be found negligent on these grounds. However, Lord Scarman was unhappy with this state of affairs. He noted that an individual's right to make their own decisions was a fundamental principle of common law. This patient had not had the opportunity to make a decision based on all the facts because the surgeon had withheld important information. The law of negligence was therefore inadequate to protect this important right of patients. He gave the opinion that the law should protect the patient further and he stated the principle of informed consent. He argued, as I already have done, that there might be important domestic, financial or personal factors, unknown to the surgeon, that would strongly influence the decision of the patient in the full knowledge of the possible complications of an operation. It was therefore the right of the patient to have full possession of the facts and to make their own decision about an operation, rather than have the surgeon decide on purely medical grounds.

In practice, this raises a serious dilemma for the surgeon. There undoubtedly exists a number of people of nervous disposition for whom the prospect of an operation is terrifying. Such people require a great deal of reassurance and many would refuse beneficial operations if a catalogue of all the possible complications and misadventures was explained to them. Even in those of a normal disposition, the anxiety generated by such a recital prior to a major operation may have a damaging effect. Many people would rather not know. Another problem is that of the power of suggestion. Consider this example: Fifty patients are told that a possible complication of a certain procedure is severe headache. A second fifty patients have this information withheld. It is commonly observed in this type of situation that following the procedure, a significantly larger number of patients in the first group will have headache, than in the second group. In other words, mentioning a complication may, by the power of suggestion, even increase the chances of that complication occurring!

There is also the difficulty of obtaining informed consent from patients who are confused, who speak a different language, who are mentally retarded or where an operation is needed with extreme urgency.

CONSENT IN PRACTICE

Unfortunately, the current British practice is to largely ignore the problem and hope it will go away. In my experience, consent to operation is rarely fully informed. The Americans, with the constant threat of litigation, have gone to the other extreme and the obtaining of consent is an elaborate affair, often involving a document of many pages setting out all the possible complications.

One of the major problems of obtaining consent from patients is that the task is delegated by the surgeon to the most junior and inexperienced doctor on the team. Even if that doctor is fully aware of what the operation entails and all the possible complications, discussing these with the patient may be taken as criticism of his senior colleagues. Any junior doctor who goes around 'upsetting' patients by suggesting that things may go wrong when his consultant does an operation will soon find himself in trouble. This is a very tricky situation for the junior doctor whose only realistic option is to avoid mentioning complications altogether. Other difficulties arise when the consultant has chosen to disguise a diagnosis, such as cancer, from the patient, referring merely to a 'blockage' that needs to be by-passed. How then is the junior doctor supposed to explain what the operation involves? How does he answer the patient's question: 'Will the operation make me better, doctor?' Even if explanations have been given, these often include medical jargon that the patient cannot understand.

The true extent of the problem was demonstrated by a survey published in the British Medical Journal in March 1988. Three researchers at the University of Dundee questioned one hundred patients a few days after their operations. Twenty-seven patients didn't know which organ of their body was operated on and forty-four were unaware of the exact nature of the surgical procedure! The level of ignorance was significantly higher in the older patients and perhaps some of these chose not to know the details of their operations, preferring to leave all decisions to the surgeon.

The current practice in obtaining consent is mirrored in the Consent Form. The usual format is as follows:

CONSENT BY THE PATIENT

..................Hospital

I ....(full name) of ....(address) hereby consent to undergo the operation of ....
....
the nature and purpose of which have been explained to me by Dr/Mr ....

I also consent to such further or alternative operative measures as may be found to be necessary during the course of the operation and to the administration of a general, local or other anaesthetic for any of these purposes.

No assurance has been given to me that the operation/procedure will be performed or administered by any particular practitioner.

Date .... (signed) ....

(patient)

I confirm that I have explained to the patient the nature and purpose of this operation.

Date .... (signed) ....

(physician/surgeon)

(The declarations of the patient and physician or surgeon should be completed concurrently)

In the light of modern attitudes and legal opinion, discussed above, I believe this form of consent is unacceptable. What it literally means is that while you lie unconscious under an anaesthetic, any surgeon can perform any operation of his choosing without consulting you further, provided he can find some medical 'justification' for the procedure. The unexpected operation might even cause disfigurement or prevent you having children. In practice, surgeons very rarely abuse this position of trust but for the reasons discussed earlier, a surgeon acting in good faith may still act against the wishes of his patient. A topical example is that of a young woman who consented to removal of a small breast lump. At operation, the surgeon discovered what was almost certainly a small breast cancer and so he removed the whole breast (mastectomy). The woman sued the surgeon on the ground that firstly, she had not given her explicit consent to mastectomy, and secondly, that this was not necessarily the best treatment for a small breast cancer. There were alternative methods of treatment such as radiotherapy that might have the same chance of cure without a disfiguring operation.

In my opinion, such a consent form should only be used in the

98 · Consent to Operation

emergency situation where an exploratory operation is required to make the diagnosis. In cases of severe internal bleeding or peritonitis, it is impossible to predict what the exact cause will be or what operation will be required once the abdomen is opened. In this case, consent is obtained for laparotomy (exploratory opening of the abdomen) with the patient's understanding that whatever further procedure is necessary will be done.

For an elective (planned) operation, there can be no justification for such a consent form. If there is any doubt in the surgeon's mind about what he may find at operation, or what course the operation will take, then he should personally discuss it with the patient. Consent should be obtained for the various possibilities after discussion with the patient and the same, named surgeon should perform the operation. If there is an unexpected finding at operation requiring a different operation then in these days of very safe anaesthesia it might sometimes be reasonable to perform a second anaesthetic and operation after discussing it with the patient. This all depends on the type of operation. The advantage of fully informed consent may be outweighed by having two relatively major operations rather than one.

So what are you to do in practice when the junior doctor asks you to sign the consent form? I would give you the following advice:

Altering the consent form

If you have no wish to know the details of your operation and are perfectly happy to leave all the decisions to the surgeon, then simply sign the consent form as it is. There is nothing wrong with doing this and very many people will feel the same way. However, if you wish to give informed consent and take an active part in decision making about your treatment, then you should protect yourself against the excessive licence given to the surgeon by the consent form. This form may be altered in any way you like. I would make the following alterations:

1. I would cross out 'such further or alternative operative measures as may be found to be necessary during the course of the operation' but would leave my consent to an anaesthetic.

2. I would find out which of the surgeons might be performing the operation and in place of the 'No assurance has been given me' paragraph, I would write: 'I understand that the operation will be performed by Mr Smith or Mr Jones' (or whatever their names might be).

Finally, I would not sign the consent form until I had discussed the operation with one of the named surgeons and I would obtain their signature on the bottom of the form.

These points require a little further explanation. What would happen if something went wrong during an operation causing danger to your life?

Would the surgeon refuse to extend the operation to cope with this situation because you have altered the consent form? The answer is a very clear 'No'. If any patient is seriously in danger the surgeon will do whatever is necessary without the patient's consent unless the patient has expressly forbidden that action. The surgeon is on very firm ground in these circumstances and could not be sued for lack of consent. Indeed, he is more likely to be sued for negligence if he failed to correct a serious problem in these circumstances. The very special case in which a patient refuses a blood transfusion is discussed later.

The right to choose your surgeon?
Do you have the right to choose which surgeon performs your operation in the NHS? The answer is 'No'. Almost always it will be one of the surgeons on the consultant's firm, of varying rank and experience. Working out who is who can be confusing and it is often not made clear which surgeon will actually perform the operation. You cannot assume that your operation will be performed by the consultant under whose name you are booked into the hospital. If you have read chapter four about the hospital staff, you will find it easier to sort out the different surgeons. Although you cannot choose your surgeon, it is reasonable to ask who is going to perform the operation. In general, major operations are carried out by senior surgeons and minor operations by junior surgeons, often under supervision.

Are you making trouble for yourself?
Will I cause trouble by insisting that one of the surgeons who is likely to be performing the operation explains the procedure to me and obtains my consent? What happens if I don't see him before the operation?

This should not be a problem in practice. Surgeons take a very direct responsibility for their work and will not perform an operation on a patient they haven't seen themselves, unless perhaps they have been seen by one of their colleagues with whom they work closely. Usually the surgeon who is actually performing the operation will come and see the patient beforehand. The consultant will often see his patients on the ward round and his more junior colleagues usually see patients at the end of a day's work, in the late afternoon or early evening. Thus there will almost always be an opportunity to discuss the operation fully and this is the appropriate time to sign the consent form, modified as necessary.

Never be afraid to ask about anything you don't understand or about which you are unhappy. You will never cause offence by asking and most surgeons are only too happy to explain an operation to you. After all, they find their work exciting and interesting and like talking about it! A common fault of doctors in general is the use of medical jargon when talking to the lay person. Do stop and ask if you don't understand a term. Throughout this book I have tried to explain things without using jargon, and where necessary, to translate jargon into plain English. At the end of the book you will find a glossary of common medical terms to help you decipher the doctor's talk.

SPECIAL SITUATIONS FOR WHICH CONSENT IS REQUIRED

Sterilisation and vasectomy

One type of operation has such profound implications for patient's lives and is such a medico-legal minefield when things go wrong, that even in this country, informed consent is carefully obtained. This type of operation is for sterilisation or vasectomy. If you have either of these operations, then a special consent form is used which is more detailed and explicit. The consent form for sterilisation of a woman has the same format and content as the standard consent form shown earlier but in addition has the following:

> 'I have been told that the intention of the operation is to render me sterile and incapable of parenthood. I understand that it may not be possible later to reverse the effect of the operation.
>
> I appreciate that the procedure involves an operation on the fallopian tubes and that the operation does not affect the ovaries or stop the period.
>
> I also appreciate that a subsequent pregnancy is most unlikely but that no operation can be guaranteed to be 100% certain preventing further children.
>
> I also consent to such further and alternative'. . .

and so on. It continues:

Date .... (signed) ....
(patient)

I confirm that I have explained to the patient the nature, purpose and effect of this operation.

Date .... (signed) ....
(physician/surgeon)

AGREEMENT BY SPOUSE
I ....(full name)
of...................................(address)
the husband of .... have read the above consent signed by my wife and hereby agree to the operation of .... being carried out on my wife, the nature, purpose and effect of which has been explained to me by Dr/Mr ....

Date .... (signed) ....
(husband)

I confirm that I have explained to the patient's husband the nature, purpose and effect of this operation.

Date .... (signed) ....
(physician/surgeon)

This consent form is a vast improvement on the standard form although it is disappointing to see the 'further or alternative measures' paragraph still remains. In this case, this clause presents very little hazard to the patient because the operation is so limited. There is very little chance of the surgeon finding anything else wrong, or wishing to do anything about it.

If a woman is of childbearing age, then other major gynaecological operations such as hysterectomy (removal of the womb) or oophorectomy (removal of the ovaries) will effectively cause sterilisation, although that is not the primary purpose. In this case, consent should be obtained with the same care, both from the patient and the spouse.

Abortion

The usual consent form for termination of pregnancy is no better than the standard form, differing simply in having the name of the operation printed rather than left as a space for the doctor to fill in. This procedure is another potential medico-legal minefield and most doctors will take care to obtain consent carefully, with explanation of the possible complications made to the patient and recorded in the case-notes. One difficulty is that the consultant gynaecologist who sees the woman in the outpatient clinic, and agrees to an abortion, rarely performs the operation. Usually, this is performed by a registrar who may only meet the patient minutes before the operation and in that time, obtain consent. I have seen a number of women who have changed their mind about abortion in these circumstances, when they are told of all the possible complications for the first time.

Minors

A person under the age of sixteen cannot legally give consent to an operation and this responsibility falls on the parent or legal guardian. A modified version of the standard consent form is used and my earlier remarks apply equally to this form.

Refusal to have a blood transfusion

Usually for religious reasons (for example Jehovah's witness), some patients refuse to accept transfusion of blood or plasma even if such refusal places their lives at risk. In ordinary circumstances a doctor will over rule the wishes of a patient in carrying out a procedure to save life. However, if the patient is determined to adhere to his or her belief even to the extent of refusing a life saving blood transfusion, then that wish will be respected. A special consent form is used, setting out the patient's wishes and absolving the doctor and hospital of any liability arising out of their refusal to consent to blood transfusion. Fortunately, even in cases of very severe blood loss, it is usually possible to preserve life by supporting the circulation with other fluids and by intensive care measures. Severe haemorrhage during a routine operation is very unusual so there is rarely a serious problem except in emergency cases.

Clinical research

Occasionally, patients in hospital for an operation are asked to volunteer for inclusion in a clinical trial. This may involve some sort of extra monitoring or measurement of your condition, before, during or after your operation. Sometimes researchers are trying to compare two slightly different operations for the same complaint, or else compare two different drugs such as pain-killers to see which is best. These trials form the scientific basis of all modern advances in medicine and surgery and no new technique or drug is accepted until it has been tested in this way. Such research may take place in any hospital, but most of it occurs in the large teaching hospitals connected with universities.

Because the research is not of direct benefit to the patient and because it may cause some discomfort or inconvenience to the patient, subjects are entered on a strictly voluntary basis. Trials cannot take place until approval has been given by the hospital ethical committee. This committee of senior doctors and lay members studies the proposed trial to make sure no harm will come to patients and that the trial is of real scientific value.

No patient can be entered into a trial without their consent and no patient should feel under any obligation to give this consent. If you wish to help the progress of medical science then the researchers will be duly grateful, but no one will mind if you refuse and your own treatment will not suffer as a result. You may benefit from participation in a clinical trial because more care is taken with your treatment and records.

SUMMARY

- A doctor cannot do anything without your consent, whether written or verbal. He may not examine you, perform a blood test or do an operation.
- You give your consent only on the understanding of the special relationship between the patient and doctor. The doctor owes you a duty of care,

he must carry out his work to a reasonable professional standard and he must maintain confidentiality.
- You have the right to be fully informed about the nature, effects and possible complications of an operation and the doctor must provide this information if you desire it. You will then be able to make your own decision about the operation.
- The present standard consent form is outdated and gives the surgeon too much licence to carry out procedures without first consulting you. It is perfectly acceptable to alter the consent form according to my suggestions or your own requirements.
- Having said all this, there is nothing wrong with avoiding all discussion of the operation and simply leaving all decisions to the surgeon. This is still what most people do and usually they are perfectly satisfied with the results.

8 The Day of Operation

SUSAN'S OPERATION

Susan woke at six in the morning and with a sudden lurch of her stomach realised this was the day of her operation. The ward clattered into life around her. She heard quick stepping footfalls, the swish of curtains, the clang of bedpans, muttered groans and the soft cajoling voices of the nurses. At seven they came to prepare her for the operation. There was time for a quick bath, they said, and then could she please put on the theatre gown, a thin cotton garment, gaping at the rear. Take off your pants and bra she was told. A draught blew through the open rear of the gown and she felt naked and undignified. She climbed back into bed and watched the other patients eating breakfast. 'NIL BY MOUTH' said the notice on the end of her bed.

At seven-thirty she was given a tablet with a little sip of water. It seemed to have no effect until they asked her to climb onto the theatre trolley when her legs felt wobbly and unco-ordinated. She felt a strange sense of calm although she knew she ought to be frightened. The theatre trolley was brought to the ward by a whistling porter dressed in green pyjamas and a blue cloth hat.

'Nice day for an operation, my love!' he said in a cheerful way.

Feeling half naked again, Susan shuffled over from the bed onto the trolley and was tucked up with blankets. The nurse from the ward did the pre-op check list.

'Can I see your identity band?. . . Susan Williams, born 12/2/54?' she confirmed, reading from the band around Susan's wrist.

'Have you eaten or drunk anything since midnight?'

'No, only the water with the tablets,' replied Susan. The consent form was inspected.

'You're having a cholecystectomy?'

'A gall-bladder operation,' said Susan.

'Yes, that's the same thing. Any contact lenses? Any dentures?'

'No,' said Susan.

'Any caps or crowns on the teeth? Any loose teeth?' Susan shook her head.

'Has the doctor marked the site of operation?. . . No, of course not, you've only one gall-bladder, they can't take out the wrong one.' Susan didn't think this was very funny.

'We've got to check, you know.'

They left the ward and turned down the corridor, the porter pulling the trolley and the ward nurse steering it at Susan's head end.

'Don't you worry,' said the nurse, 'I'll stay with you until you're asleep.' Why don't they repaint the grimy ceilings, thought Susan.

At the entrance to the theatre suite, they paused alongside another trolley. The porter inserted two long poles down each side of a canvas sheet beneath Susan, to form a stretcher. Another man came out of the theatre and took the place of the porter.

'Hello, my dear. We're just going to lift you over onto the other trolley.' He checked Susan's identity bracelet and consent form and led the trolley into one of the anaesthetic rooms down the corridor. The corridor seemed full of busy people, all wearing green uniforms, hats and masks. The decor was shiny pale green with stainless steel fittings. The doors on either side had round glass port-holes.

After the bustle of the corridor, the anaesthetic room seemed quiet and peaceful. A set of double doors led through into the operating theatre from where Susan could hear the muffled sounds of voices and of instruments being laid out in preparation. Susan noticed for the first time that the nurse had put a green gown over her uniform and had covered her hair with a hat.

The room was brightly lit and functional. In one corner, behind her head, was a machine with lots of pipes, hoses, dials, knobs, chrome fittings and gas cylinders. Along the walls were cupboards and shelves full of drugs, syringes, needles, drip sets and other equipment. A clear, polythene bag of fluid hung from a tall stand at Susan's side, connected to a narrow plastic tube. The hand basin next to the door had long chrome levers on the taps. The door opened and Dr Lewis, the anaesthetist, came in. Susan recognised him from his visit to the ward the evening before.

'Hello, Susan, how are you feeling?' he said over his shoulder as he washed his hands. 'This is my ODA who helps with the anaesthetic,' indicating the man who had collected Susan from the theatre entrance.

'Peter,' turning to him, 'I'll be doing a thoracic epidural at the beginning so we'll take her through and do it on the operating table when we've got the monitors on.'

The nurse squeezed Susan's arm below the elbow and asked her to open and close her fist.

'Gets the veins standing up,' said Dr Lewis. 'I'll just get the drugs ready.' Susan could hear him snapping open glass ampoules and watched him fill several syringes. Each one he carefully labelled.

Feeling for a vein just above her wrist he warned, 'A sharp prick and sting,' as he made a small injection of local anaesthetic into the skin over the vein. In a few seconds it was numb and Susan felt no pain when the much bigger needle of the drip was put in her arm. This was connected to the tubing from the bag of fluid and she could feel the cold liquid passing up her arm. To Susan's surprise, he showed her a large needle saying, 'That's the needle. I've taken it out. All you've got is a tiny plastic tube going into the vein and it can't hurt you or cut you so you can quite safely move your arm.'

While this was going on, the ODA had loosened the gown behind Susan's neck and put self adhesive electrodes on her chest. 'That's to measure your heart beat while you're asleep.' He wrapped a blood pressure cuff around her arm and strapped a thin metal foil plate to her thigh.

'What's that for,' asked Susan.

'That's the earthing plate for the diathermy machine which the surgeon uses to seal off small blood vessels and stop the bleeding.'

Dr Lewis took one of the syringes and plugged the tip into an injection port on the drip on Susan's wrist.

'This is some pain-killer, first of all. It might make you feel rather tipsy.' The nurse held her hand and felt her pulse. Susan couldn't feel the injection going in but suddenly felt pleasantly woozy.

'This is the one to put you to sleep,' and plugging a second syringe into the drip, he gradually began to inject. 'Take a big breath'.

And that was the last thing Susan remembered before waking up in a different room. . .

She woke to the sound of her name being called.

'Susan!. . . Susan, wake up! Your operation's finished.' She recognised the voice of Dr Lewis and opened her eyes but was dazzled by a bright light. She closed them again.

'All right, staff?' said Dr Lewis to the nurse watching over Susan. 'I'll go and start my second case then,' in response to her nod. His footsteps receded and Susan opened her eyes again. The first thing she noticed was a clock on the wall. She was astonished to find the time was only nine forty-five. She had woken as if from a deep sleep and felt as if a much longer time had passed. She looked around and found herself in a room divided into a number of bays, each with a patient on a trolley, and an attendant nurse. In each bay there was apparatus for administering oxygen, a suction device, an angle-poise lamp, a blood pressure scale and what she took to be a heart monitor. Several were switched on and emitted soft, regular beeps.

The nurse looking after Susan counted her pulse, checked her blood pressure and measured her temperature. She recorded the numbers on a chart on the end of Susan's trolley. Susan became aware of a soreness in her nose and an uncomfortable feeling of something stuck in the back of her throat. Swallowing made the feeling worse. Feeling with her hand she discovered a plastic tube coming out of her nostril, secured with some sticky tape.

'Try not to pull it, Susan,' said the nurse, 'We'll take it out in a short while.' Susan later learnt that this was a nasogastric tube which went right down her throat into her stomach. Its purpose was to keep the stomach completely empty and to drain out any bile which accumulated in the stomach during the operation. The free end was connected to a plastic bag which contained a small amount of the bitter green liquid. Some patients, like George, who are having major abdominal surgery need a nasogastric tube for several days. Susan was relieved when the tube was pulled out half an hour later. It came quite easily but made her gag slightly and the back of her head stung like the feeling of getting salt water up the nose when swimming.

'Does your tummy hurt?' asked the nurse. Susan noticed with surprise the absence of any sensation from her tummy and wondered for a moment if the operation had actually been performed. Feeling with her hand she discovered that most of her tummy was rather numb but there was a definite line of tenderness in the midline above her tummy button. She shook her head.

'The epidural's working nicely then,' said the nurse. Susan found she could move on the trolley without causing much discomfort. As she moved she felt a pulling on the skin of her shoulder. This was the epidural cannula, a plastic tube only a millimetre in diameter, which emerged from her back between the shoulder blades and was taped to the skin up and over her right shoulder. The tube terminated in a syringe attached to a slim box slightly smaller than a paperback book. A small indicator lamp flashed at regular intervals as minute doses of pain-killer were fed into the epidural tube. The device was battery powered and the syringe contained enough drug to last for two days, providing continuous pain relief.

'Can I have a drink?' asked Susan.

'Just a sip or it'll make you feel sick. You're getting plenty of fluid in the drip but I'll give you a little to freshen your mouth.'

Now that Susan was well awake and the nurse was satisfied with her observations, she could return to her ward. Her trolley was pushed to the door. Poles were inserted once more into the canvas and she was lifted onto another trolley. A nurse from her ward appeared and together with a porter they wheeled her along the same route back to the ward.

'Why do I have to keep changing trolleys?' asked Susan.

'Well, they've got special trolleys in theatre,' said the porter. 'They've got oxygen cylinders and cot-sides and they can tip head down in case a patient is sick. This is just an ordinary ward trolley. And besides, the ward trolleys can't go into theatre because they've got dirty wheels. Just like we have to change into special clean shoes if we go into theatre.'

Reaching the ward, Susan was lifted onto what she thought was the wrong bed but looking up, she found her name on the frame.

'We always put post-op patients in beds near the nurse's desk. Then we can keep an eye on you. As you get better, we'll move your bed further down the ward again and other patients who have just had their operation will be put here.'

GEORGE'S OPERATION

As George's operation wasn't until the afternoon, he was allowed a cup of tea at seven o'clock in the morning. Other patients who were having minor operations in the afternoon were allowed some light breakfast but George was having special treatment to empty his bowels. The houseman explained why this was necessary.

'When we do your operation, we have to cut out a segment of your large bowel where the tumour is. Then we have to join the cut ends together again. If we don't have the bowel completely empty and clean, the bacteria in the faeces could cause a very serious infection which would stop the healing process. Also we want the bowel to rest because any activity could put a strain on the stitches where the join is made. The best way of giving the bowel a rest is to make sure that it's completely empty. That's also why we won't be letting you eat anything for five days after the operation.'

Getting the bowel empty was not the most pleasant experience for George. They started the day before with a low-residue diet. Then he was given a powerful laxative in the form of a white powder dissolved in water. The effect of this was explosive and poor George spent much of the afternoon on the toilet with profuse diarrhoea. A repeat dose the next morning, on an empty stomach, was almost more than he could bear. George felt weak and shaky. The final indignity was an enema late in the morning. He was asked to lie on his side on the bed. Using some lubricating jelly, the nurse gently inserted a rubber tube into his bottom. George kept feeling as if he was about to soil himself but the nurse reassured him that the feeling was due to the tube and that he wasn't making any mess. Using a funnel, she gently poured warm soapy liquid into the tube and then let it run out again into a bucket. She repeated this several times until the liquid came back clean. George was intensely embarrassed to have these ministrations performed on the ward, just behind thin curtains, but at least there wasn't any smell.

Although George's operation was being done by the same surgeon, there was a different anaesthetist for the afternoon list, Dr Johnson. Like Dr Lewis, he had visited the ward the evening before. From experience, he knew that the laxatives could cause severe dehydration in some patients and this could cause problems during the anaesthetic and operation, resulting in low blood pressure. For this reason, when he saw George in the evening, he inserted a drip in his arm and prescribed several bags of saline (salt and water solution) to replace what George lost in the diarrhoea. Dr Johnson was not much in favour of epidurals although he used them for certain selected cases. Unlike

Susan, George would be having a cut in the lower half of the tummy and this was not as painful as one at the top of the tummy which moves with each breath. For a major operation, Dr Johnson liked to use a much stronger pre-med so, just after midday, George was given an injection rather than a tablet. This contained a mixture of powerful pain-killer and a sedative which also had an anti-emetic action (prevents nausea and vomiting). By the time the porter came to collect George for his operation, he was very drowsy and sedated and he later had no clear recollection of the rest of that day. As he already had a drip in his arm, it was a simple matter to put him to sleep with an injection into the drip.

After his operation, he was transferred to the recovery ward like Susan but stayed there for some hours. He had had a much longer operation and heavier anaesthetic and so was slower to wake up. Also, to make sure he would be comfortable post-operatively, he was given further doses of pain-killer before the end of his operation. This made him very drowsy and rather disorientated. If he was disturbed, he became aware of a constant ache in his stomach and also of shivering intensely. Most of the time, though, he slept. The shivering was partly a side effect of the anaesthetic and partly because he had lost heat on the operating table. Dr Johnson was well aware of the problem. During such a major operation, a large area of wet bowel is exposed to the atmosphere and evaporation causes considerable heat loss, rather like the way a damp cloth is chilled by a breeze. Every possible precaution was taken to minimise heat loss. George was placed on an electrically heated mattress on the operating table. All fluids and blood going into the drip were warmed to body temperature as they were infused. All exposed parts of his body were covered as much as possible. None the less George's temperature had dropped during the operation and in the recovery ward he was wrapped in a foil space blanket. Because shivering involves a lot of muscular activity, this increased George's oxygen consumption. In combination with the slowing of breathing caused by the pain-killers, the shivering could potentially lead to an oxygen shortage but this was easily prevented by giving extra oxygen with a face mask, back on the ward. Although George wasn't aware, the mask was kept in place all night as he slept.

JOHN'S OPERATION

John was the only patient not visited by the anaesthetist because he was having the operation under local anaesthetic, usually administered by the surgeon. Like the others, he had been starved on the day of operation. Although this is not strictly necessary for a local anaesthetic, patients are always starved in case the local anaesthetic is inadequate and a general anaesthetic is required. (A very unusual occurrence.) Instead of going into the anaesthetic room he was wheeled into the operating theatre awake. Like Susan, heart-beat and blood pressure monitors were attached to him and the diathermy earthing plate strapped to his leg. While all this was going on, the surgeon put a small needle in a vein on the back of John's hand.

John had a paroxysm of coughing and had to ask for a tissue to spit out the phlegm. He began to feel breathless lying flat and so when he was lifted over onto the operating table, the head of the table was tilted to lift his head and chest. He was given oxygen to breathe with a special mask that didn't restrict his breathing and which provided a controlled amount of oxygen. Paradoxically, too much oxygen could actually be harmful for John. His lung condition was so bad that his brain had adapted itself to a low oxygen concentration, and if too much was given when he was sedated, his brain could be confused into thinking he didn't need to breathe any more.

'Mr Reynolds, I'm going to give you something now to make you feel very relaxed and sleepy,' said Mr Brown as he injected a small amount of a sleeping drug into the needle. 'It won't put you right out to sleep and you'll still be able to talk. I don't mind if you cough but please warn me beforehand otherwise I might cut the wrong piece of tissue.' John could appreciate this because he knew the hernia moved in and out when he coughed. Indeed, it was the chronic cough that had partly caused the hernia.

As the drug was injected, John began to feel pleasantly woozy and all his feelings of apprehension vanished. He watched with a detached interest as all the preparations were made for surgery. After checking the consent form and inspecting the skin for the ink-drawn arrow marking the site of the operation, the surgeon stepped through a doorway into the scrub room. Here John could see him washing his hands with disinfectant, right up to the elbows. The hands and nails were scrubbed with a sterile scrubbing brush and the soaping and rinsing repeated before the hands were carefully dried on sterile towels. John admired the way the surgeon donned the sterile gown and gloves without touching any of the outside surfaces. He was already wearing a hat and mask. The surgeon's assistant, who this morning was the senior house officer, likewise scrubbed and gowned.

A bar was fitted over John's lower chest so that when it was draped with a sheet, it would form a screen, blocking John's view of the surgery. A theatre nurse, who had scrubbed earlier, laid out all the surgical instruments on a sterile tray. She painted a wide area of skin around the groin with a pink antiseptic solution, to clean the skin. Then, together with the surgeon, a series of sterile green sheets was laid over his legs and abdomen such that only the area of the hernia remained bare.

'Mr Reynolds, we're ready to start the operation now so I'm going to start injecting the local anaesthetic. With each injection, you'll feel a sharp prick and then some stinging. Then it'll quickly go numb.' Using his knowledge of the anatomy, the surgeon was able to place injections so that the three main nerves supplying the groin region were blocked in turn. John could feel the needle going in and out and although he knew in a theoretical sort of way that this was a painful sensation, the effect of the sedative drug was to produce such a relaxed frame of mind that he really didn't mind at all.

'There's a deeper part of the tissues that I'll have to inject half way through the operation but the rest should be completely numb by now. Just let me know if it hurts at any stage.'

'Fine,' said John.

'I've started the actual operation now.' All John could feel was the pressure of the surgeon's wrist leaning on his upper leg. He began to feel more drowsy and fell into a light sleep. . .

He was roused when they lifted him back onto a trolley from the operating table.

'When are you going to do my operation?' he said.

'It's all finished, Mr Reynolds.' John shook his head in bewilderment. He had no recollection of any of the operation.

'I thought you weren't going to give me an anaesthetic,' he said.

'We didn't,' said the surgeon. 'You were quite awake when we started the operation but you probably can't remember because the sedative I gave you has very strong amnesic properties.' John still found it hard to believe the operation had been done but when he looked at the clock, he realised that nearly an hour had passed. There was no pain or discomfort at the operation site but over the next few hours, as the local anaesthetic wore off, it became increasingly uncomfortable. However, some simple paracetamol tablets relieved most of the pain and John declined any stronger pain-killers.

BETTY'S OPERATION

Betty was last on the morning operating list. She was given a simple pre-med tablet, like Susan, and dozed much of the morning. She didn't feel at all sleepy when she saw Dr Lewis in the anaesthetic room but at least the anxiety of a long wait had been eased. Dr Lewis had found her to be a cheerful and phlegmatic character on his pre-op visit and so had judged a strong pre-med unnecessary. He deftly inserted a very small needle into a vein on the back of her hand.

'Mrs Johnson, I'll ask the surgeon to inject some local anaesthetic into the two main cuts, so you shouldn't be in too much discomfort when you wake up. That'll last about six or eight hours.'

'Oh! Doctor, you're so thoughtful. Everyone's been so kind. I think you're all wonderful.' She squeezed the hand of the nurse who had accompanied her from the ward, and smiled.

112 · The Day of Operation

Dr Lewis approached her with a large syringe full of a milky white drug. 'This is the one to put you to sleep. We call it "Milk of Amnesia"!' he said in a joking manner. It's a very nice anaesthetic. No hangover, you wake up very quickly and you won't feel sick at all. The only problem is, sometimes it stings a bit in the vein when I inject it. Not too bad really.'

Betty felt drowsy and began to day-dream. She gave a huge yawn. She was still dreaming about her husband, Bill, when she gradually became aware of a different voice calling.

'Oh! You are lovely, darling. . .' She held Bill's hand and then, coming further to her senses, realised that in fact she held Dr Lewis's hand as she was wheeled down the corridor to the recovery ward.

'Your operation's finished, Mrs Johnson. Everything's gone very well.'

'How embarrassing! What have I been saying? I was having such a nice dream.'

'Not to worry. I've never yet discovered anyone's secrets!'

They parked in one of the bays in the recovery ward and Dr Lewis greeted the nurse who immediately joined him.

'Hello, Sue. How are you? This is Betty Johnson, forty-eight, a fit lady who's had bilateral varicose veins. She's had injections of Bupivicaine in both the groin incisions so she should be fairly comfortable. I've written her up for a stat dose of omnopon if she needs it but I expect she'll be all right with some paracetamol. OK?'

About half an hour later, Betty was taken back to her ward. By that time she'd discovered the names and ages of Sue's children and was inviting them for a day out on the farm!

TUBES AND THINGS

The further progress of our four patients is followed in the next chapter. One aspect of the early post-operative recovery that tends to frighten and confuse patients is the number of drips and tubes they wake up with. In fact these are all perfectly simple to understand and are not nearly as bad as they look. So that you can follow what happens in the next few days, I'll explain now about four common types of tube, all of which George has: the drip, nasogastric tube, surgical drain, and the urinary catheter.

Drips

We learnt how a drip was inserted when Susan had her anaesthetic. They come in various brands and sizes but all have the common feature of insertion with a needle which is then withdrawn, leaving only a fine plastic tube (cannula) in the vein. Drips are used for several purposes: to administer fluids to someone who isn't drinking, to give a blood transfusion, or to administer intravenous drugs such as antibiotics. The bag or bottle of fluid is connected to the cannula by a clear plastic tube which has a drip chamber near the top. The rate of flow is adjusted by a small clamp on the tube such that a certain number of drips form per second. If accurate control of the flow is required, a machine is connected to the tube which counts the drips and automatically adjusts the rate.

There are a number of problems with drips which will occupy the houseman both day and night. The presence of foreign material in the vein causes an inflammatory reaction which limits the life of any one drip. After one or two days, the drip site will start to become swollen and tender and eventually the vein will thrombose (formation of blood clot) and the flow will stop. A new drip will then have to be inserted in a different vein. If this is done at an early stage, the vein will recover. Otherwise, the blockage becomes permanent and this segment of the vein will shrink into a fibrous band. This is not harmful in itself as the veins form a complex network with many alternative paths. However, the successive loss of veins in a patient requiring longer term intravenous therapy can be a problem.

Anaesthetists often use local anaesthetic when inserting the larger drips but the doctors on the ward usually put in a smaller drip without local. If deftly done, the pain is sharp but momentary; it does not hurt once it is in place.

A drip placed on the back of the wrist tends to be temperamental. When the wrist is cocked back, the flow stops by a valve-like action and for this reason, the wrist is sometimes splinted with a board to keep it in the best position.

Two occurrences tend to worry patients. The first is the sight of blood coming back into the drip tubing. This happens most often when the drip is turned off or the flow is obstructed for some reason. There is nothing to be alarmed about and no harm can be done. Usually just a simple adjustment is needed. Even if the drip cannula was accidentally pulled right out of your arm, the blood loss would be slight before the vein sealed itself. The other concern is the sight of an air bubble passing down the tube into the arm. Again, this is quite harmless unless a large quantity of air was injected in this way. As a precaution against this, intravenous fluids are presented in airtight bags which collapse when empty and no air can enter the system.

A drip need not necessarily tie you to the bed. The drip stand from which the bag of fluid hangs is usually mounted on castor wheels. Provided you are otherwise mobile and have sought the advice of a doctor or nurse, there is no reason why you can't walk the drip stand with you and visit the bathroom, for instance. This becomes much more difficult if you have more than one drip, like George. He has one to provide fluids, and a separate one for regular doses of intravenous antibiotics.

Finally, a word about a special sort of drip called a central venous line. This is a drip with a much longer cannula that reaches into one of the great veins in the chest. It is inserted under fully aseptic conditions and is often stitched in place. Usually these are placed on the side of the neck or just under the collar bone. Looked after carefully, they can last for weeks or months. They are used for a variety of specialised purposes including total intravenous feeding which can replace a normal diet. Mostly, they are found on patients in intensive care units but also occasionally on the general surgical ward.

Nasogastric tubes

These tubes are passed through the nose, down the back of the throat and into the stomach. They are used either to drain the stomach artificially, or to provide a route for a liquid diet in someone who has difficulty eating. They come in a wide variety of sizes and materials and the most comfortable are the fine-bore feeding tubes made of a very soft silicone rubber. Anyone having a major operation involving the stomach or gut is likely to wake up from the anaesthetic with one of these in place. Why are they needed?

If the abdomen is opened during an operation, and the bowel handled or cut, it tends to go on strike. The waves of muscular contraction that normally propel food along the bowel are inhibited and as a result, fluid and gas tends to accumulate within the bowel and stomach. This is particularly likely to happen if morphine-like pain-killers are given because they have a direct inhibitory action on the bowels, causing constipation. This condition, technically known as an ileus, has several consequences. Bloating of the stomach can cause nausea and vomiting and the patient may also suffer considerable discomfort from wind. If the whole abdomen becomes distended, this can put a strain on the stitches. Finally, if a join has been made in the bowel, undue stress may be placed on the join before it has a chance to heal. A nasogastric tube allows free drainage of gas and fluid and prevents any accumulation.

'When will I be allowed to drink?' asks George. When the bowel starts working again, is the answer. When the doctors visited George on their morning ward round the second day after his operation, the houseman listened to his abdomen with a stethoscope. He was listening for the rumbling sounds that bowel makes when it is active.

'Passed any wind yet, Mr Saunders?' asked the registrar. With confirmation of both signs that the ileus had resolved, they said he could begin drinking cautiously. The 'NIL BY MOUTH' sign on the end of George's bed was changed to '30 ML PER HOUR'. Each hour, a nurse poured him the measured amount into a small beaker. George was allowed to sip this slowly and at the end of each hour, the nurse sucked on the nasogastric tube with a syringe. If the stomach was now working, it would empty itself and no fluid would come up the nasogastric tube. If the stomach was still on strike, the water would be detected by this aspiration test and the drinking would be stopped again. Over the next twenty-four hours, increasing hourly amounts were allowed with checks at each stage. The next day he was permitted to satisfy his thirst with clear fluids, and the drip was discontinued.

There is one further use for a nasogastric tube. If during the operation, a join has been made in the oesophagus (gullet) or stomach, then a nasogastric tube is passed through the joined passage and left in place for at least five days. This ensures that a clear passage remains as the cut ends heal together.

Wound drains

These are smooth plastic or rubber tubes, perforated at their deep end, which pass through the skin into a surgical wound. They vary in size from a few millimetres to a centimetre or more in diameter but all serve the same purpose. Any cut surface of tissue will ooze fluid and some blood until the cellular repair process takes place. In a small wound where the surgeon has been careful to stop all bleeding, this doesn't matter and the fluid will be absorbed naturally. In a larger wound, a collection of fluid can present a hazard.

Firstly, the fluid is very rich in the sort of nutrients that bacteria like. When this fluid is kept at body temperature, it forms the perfect incubator and serious infection can result. Antibiotics will not prevent this as they will not reach the fluid in significant concentrations. For similar reasons, the body's own immune system will not cope well with infection in a large fluid collection. All these problems are avoided if the fluid volume is kept small by draining through a tube.

Secondly, a collection of fluid will keep tissue planes apart and prevent them being knitted together in the healing process. A tense collection of fluid can also be quite painful.

Most drains are put in along the line of a wound, lying in the tissues below the skin. George has one like this but also has a much larger one going deep into his abdomen. When his operation was performed, a section of large bowel was removed, not far above the back passage. The two cut ends were then sewn back together in an awkward procedure carried out deep in the pelvis. Even in the most skilled hands, a perfect join is not always possible and sometimes a small leak develops. Any material that leaks from the bowel is always heavily contaminated with germs and may cause an abscess deep in the pelvis that will further endanger the join. This problem can be avoided if a drain is placed right down in the pelvis, near the join. Any leak is betrayed by the presence of dirty fluid coming out of the drain. Usually the situation will resolve itself if free drainage is maintained. Sometimes, the contamination can be washed away by irrigating the drain with sterile fluid, allowing it to drain out again.

All drains are connected to an airtight bag or bottle and some have simple suction devices attached. Usually the drain is fixed to the skin with a stitch. The drains stay in only until the discharge stops, usually one to three days. Removing the drains is a simple and painless matter. The stitch is cut and the drain gently pulled out. Because the drain is made of very smooth material, it doesn't adhere to any tissues. When the drain is removed, the skin puncture site may ooze a little fluid but usually this dries up in a day or two.

Urinary catheters

These are tubes that pass into the bladder and drain the urine. They are made of soft rubber or plastic and are usually inserted up the urethra (outlet of urination) after the application of local anaesthetic jelly. Inside the bladder, a small balloon is inflated on the end of the catheter which prevents it falling out. The other end of the catheter is connected via a tube to a closed drainage bag. This tube is secured to the leg with elastoplast so that an accidental tug on the tube will not pull directly on your bladder. If you have a urinary catheter, it will probably be inserted while you are asleep.

A urinary catheter has two purposes. Firstly, because of the effect of the operation, it may not be possible to pass urine naturally. For instance, if you are a lady having a pelvic floor repair, the bruising and swelling around the urethra and bladder neck may temporarily obstruct the urine flow. When the swelling has diminished in a few days, the catheter would be taken out.

Secondly, in a patient having a major operation, a catheter may be used to measure accurately the hourly urine output. This is an extremely valuable indicator of the state of the circulation. Through losses of blood and various body fluids, a patient may become seriously dehydrated during an operation or illness. The diminished blood circulation affects the function of internal organs such as the liver and kidney. This is demonstrated by an immediate reduction in urine flow which can only be detected if the bladder is catheterized. During the first night after George's operation, his blood pressure began to fall and the hourly urine output dropped markedly. The houseman was called out of bed to assess the situation and after making sure there was no sign of internal bleeding, diagnosed excessive fluid loss from the drains. The drip was sped up and blood pressure and urine output returned to normal.

The catheter in place may cause some initial discomfort and, in men particularly, it causes a sensation of wanting to pass water even though the bladder is empty. This sensation usually passes after the first day. Catheters predispose to urinary infection, especially in women, and their use is therefore minimised. Older men who have enlarged prostate glands and a poor urinary stream sometimes go into acute retention of urine after an operation. The bladder becomes increasingly and painfully distended, blocking the outflow of urine by a valve like effect. The houseman will be on the look out for this and will catheterize the bladder on the ward if necessary. Usually, the patient will be able to pass urine again when he is recovered but sometimes he will be recommended for a prostate operation.

An alternative type of urinary catheter is inserted by needle through the skin above the pubis, therefore called a suprapubic catheter. This needs to be done either while a patient is asleep, or under local anaesthetic. The advantage of this type of catheter is that the urethra is left undisturbed. If the doctor wishes to find out if the patient can pass urine normally, the suprapubic catheter is clamped and the bladder allowed to fill. If the patient is unable to pass urine, the catheter is allowed to drain again. Otherwise it can be removed.

Like a surgical drain, the catheter comes out easily and painlessly. After the catheter has been in place for a few days, the passage through the tissues from the skin to the bladder becomes lined with a membrane. When the catheter is withdrawn, this membrane prevents urine from leaking into the tissues from the small hole in the bladder wall. The passage closes and heals remarkably quickly and the small leakage of urine to the skin dries up almost immediately.

9 Post-operative Recovery

The last chapter described the experiences of our four patients on the day of their operation and explained some of the technicalities of post-operative care. Now that you understand the simple principles of drips and drains and so on, we can chart the day by day progress of their recovery.

In the first few days after an operation, patients may complain of many different symptoms. Of these, pain is the one that most concerns patients and I will discuss the many different methods of pain relief. You may also experience a number of other discomforts in these days such as sore throat, wind, and muscle stiffness. Some of these are side effects of the anaesthetic, and some of having the operation itself. Each of these topics is illustrated by the story of our four characters, as are the events of post-operative care on the ward.

Surgeons like to plan care by counting days after the operation so we will do the same.

DAY ONE

George

It wasn't until the morning that George really became aware of his surroundings although he had very vague recollections of visits from a nurse in the night to check his blood pressure or adjust the drip. He woke to the sounds of the ward coming to life and became aware of the constant ache in his stomach. Whenever he moved, the pain stabbed. He didn't like to bother the busy staff but the pain gradually became worse and he began to sweat.

'Nurse!. . . Nurse!' he eventually called out. 'The pain, it's really hurting in my stomach.'

'OK Mr Saunders, I'll get you some more pain-killer in a minute. I've just got to find another nurse.' The ward was busy and it was a while before another nurse was free. Because of the strict regulations governing the use of powerful pain-killers like morphine, an injection could only be given if it was checked by two qualified nurses and recorded in the book. This inevitably leads to delays, especially at night when the second nurse might have to be called from another ward. The injection was given into his leg but the pain still became worse. Eventually, about half an hour later, the pain eased off and George was able to relax again.

'Don't be afraid to ask for a pain-killer, Mr Saunders. It never works straight away so it's best to ask for it as soon as the last dose begins to wear off. You can have an injection every four hours. If it makes you feel sick, we can give you an injection for that as well.' George had certainly learnt his lesson. He didn't want that pain again!

At eight o'clock the surgical team came onto the ward to do a quick ward-round. The senior registrar, who had performed George's operation, was accompanied by the senior house officer, the two housemen and a staff nurse. Brief progress reports were made and instructions given before moving swiftly onto the next bed.

'The operation went very well, Mr Saunders. I think we've got it all out and there was no evidence of any spread.' Turning to the houseman, enquiry was made about the urine output.

'Yes, fine! Forty ml per hour in the last few hours. I sped up the drip in the night because the urine output was falling off a bit.'

George was feeling drowsy again from the injection and spent most of the day sleeping fitfully. From time to time, a nurse came and checked the drips, drains and catheter and recorded the amounts on the chart at the end of his bed. Three times during the day and night, an infusion of antibiotics was connected to the drip. Before any medication was given, his identity was checked on the wrist-band and the hospital number checked against his charts. Every four hours, a nurse came and checked his blood pressure, pulse rate and temperature. At ten o'clock, the houseman came and took a blood sample. He explained this was a blood-count to check how much blood he had lost during the operation, and U&E to check the blood chemistry and kidney function. When the results of the tests were back from the laboratory, the houseman came back and inspected the charts. He was anxious that George should maintain a good urine output, and after studying all the figures, he calculated what fluids George would need in the drip in the next twenty-four hours.

Afterwards, George could remember little of what had happened on day one. He was not allowed anything to drink or eat and mostly the attention of the staff seemed to be on the tubes and he was not directly disturbed. When he complained that his mouth felt very dry and dirty, a nurse performed a mouth toilet using a small sponge dipped in mouth wash solution. What George remembered most was the visit of the physiotherapist, late in the morning.

An attractive young lady, dressed in navy blue trousers and a white tunic, she had visited George before his operation to teach him some breathing exercises. Her first post-operative visit was something of an ordeal. With the help of a nurse, she had propped George up on several pillows. She listened to George's chest with a stethoscope and laid her hands on his chest as he tried several deep breaths.

'I thought so!. . . Mr Saunders, I know it's painful but we really must get that chest moving better or you are going to get a chest infection.' Because of the discomfort, George had been breathing rather shallowly, and a segment of the lung just above the diaphragm was starting to collapse.

'See where my hand is? You've got to breath right down into the bottom of your chest, like I showed you before your operation. Big breath in now!' George winced. 'That's better. Try again. . . Good. Now, I want you to practise this deep breathing as often as you can. It's very important.'

'I'm going to help you with some coughing. I can hear crackles down at the left base and we need to try and shift that sputum. Place your hands flat on your tummy and press gently on the wound. When you cough, that'll take some of the strain off the wound and it won't hurt so much. Now, when I say, cough! Deep breath in. . . cough!' As George coughed, she squeezed the lower part of his chest with a juddering movement to reinforce the cough. This was repeated several times at different parts of his chest and was quite painful but he could feel his chest was easier by the end. He brought up several lumps of thick sputum and this was collected in a sterile container and sent to the laboratory to check for infection.

George began to feel exhausted and resented the bullying. 'I've just had a major operation,' he thought, 'why can't they just leave me in peace to rest.' The physiotherapist caught the expression on his face, and smiled in sympathy.

'I'm sorry, Mr Saunders. I know it's all a bit of an ordeal but it is very important for your recovery. I've nearly finished.'

'What, more?' thought George. She pulled back the bed-clothes and briefly massaged his calves.

'Have you been keeping these legs moving like I told you?' Waggling his feet up and down, she reminded him of the exercise he had forgotten.

'You must do this yourself to keep the blood flowing in your legs. If you lie still, the blood flow can stagnate and you might get a thrombosis. Wiggle your feet whenever you remember. The stockings will help but you've got to do it yourself.' George had forgotten he was wearing stockings. Before his operation, they had put surgical elasticated stockings on his legs which initially felt very tight. They were made of a white material and firmly gripped his whole foot and leg although they had a hole for the toes. They were designed to prevent pooling of blood in the veins and reduce the risk of a deep vein thrombosis. This is another important subject to be discussed later.

'Well done, Mr Saunders. I'll come and see you again tomorrow. Don't forget the exercises!'

Susan

Susan woke to the sound of a soft whirring noise in her ear. The sound came again and was mingled with the noise of the ward coming to life as Susan became aware of her strange surroundings. She had slept soundly. Like the new pupil waking after her first night at boarding school, Susan lay still in the security of her bed rather than acknowledge the uncertainties of the day ahead.

She analysed the sound in her ear and realised it was coming from the infusion pump that was delivering a steady stream of pain-killer into her epidural catheter. The pump lay on the pillow beside her. Mentally exploring her own body she was surprised to find no pain other than a bruised feeling below her ribcage on the right, and a generalised stiffness. If she moved in the bed, the wound was tender but she could breathe in comfort and an experimental deep breath was merely uncomfortable. She could clearly recall the previous day's events and remembered waking in the recovery ward after her operation. The muzzy feeling in her head that had persisted all afternoon and evening was gone. Her tummy rumbled loudly and she felt hungry.

By the time the doctors came round at 8 o'clock, she was sitting out in a chair at the side of her bed and doing yesterday's crossword.

'Hello Mrs Williams, looking very well!'

'Yes, fine thank you.'

'These epidurals are marvellous, aren't they?' The houseman nodded enthusiastically. He had been very impressed with the difference in post-operative recovery between patients with epidurals and those having ordinary pain- killing injections. Not only was the pain relief superb, but the patients were always alert and keen to get up and about.

'Operation went very well. Have you seen your gall-stones?' Susan showed him the plastic pot on her locker, containing the stones.

'We did an x-ray of the bile duct during the operation and that was all clear, with no stones stuck down there, so you shouldn't have any more trouble.'

'When can I eat? I'm starving.'

'Well, you can drink whatever you like during the day and if that's going down alright, you can start a light diet this evening. We'll take the drip out so then you won't have any tubes.'

'How long does the epidural stay in?'

'Usually forty-eight hours and by that time some simple paracetamol should be enough to keep you comfortable.'

'And how long do I have to keep these awful stockings on?'

'Well, if you're up and about tomorrow, you can take them off.'

Late in the morning the anaesthetist visited Susan to ask how the epidural was working.

'Fine! When I sit still I don't have any pain at all. My throat hurts more than my tummy.'

The physiotherapist came equally briefly. Susan saw her coming and began to take huge breaths in an exaggerated manner with a grin on her face. The physio' laughed.

'I can see that you don't need my services. Keep those feet wiggling!'

Betty

Betty went home the first day after her operation. She had been allowed to eat the evening before and had felt perfectly clear headed without any hangover effects. Her legs felt sore and very bruised but the wounds in each side of her groin were numbed with the local anaesthetic which only started to wear off as she went to bed. These spots were very tender the next morning and walking was painful with a sharp tug at each step. Both her legs were swathed in bandages which increased the feeling of stiffness. After some paracetamol she felt more comfortable and was quite OK if she settled in a chair.

Following the morning ward round, one of the surgeons returned and supervised a change of bandages. The new dressings were wrapped tightly around her legs. Before she left, she was sternly warned that her home going was conditional on strictly following advice: She was to keep her legs elevated on a stool whenever she sat down. She must do the exercises and keep her feet moving. Patients having varicose vein surgery were particularly prone to thrombosis in the legs, she was told, and these were important precautions against this complication. The bandages were not to be removed until she was seen in the clinic at the hospital in five days' time, when healing of the wounds would be checked.

John

John had a bad night and felt weary and more breathless than usual on the first morning after his operation. The previous afternoon he had been fine. The local anaesthetic was still working and he could cough without any discomfort. The physiotherapist came early in the afternoon and worked hard on his chest, clearing quite a volume of dirty sputum.

During the evening, the local anaesthetic began to wear off. John had some paracetamol and was all right until he went to bed. As so often happened, lying down provoked his coughing and he had several prolonged bouts. Each cough produced a severe pain in the wound in his groin, which left him gasping and breathless. He pushed the bell call to alert a nurse because he couldn't stand the pain any more. She helped him out of bed into an armchair where his coughing wouldn't be so bad and went to bleep

Post-operative Recovery · 123

the on call houseman. After a delay of several minutes the phone rang and she recognised the sleepy voice of Dr Peters.

'Sorry to wake you, doctor, but we're having great problems with one of the patients who's in a lot of pain.'

'Who's that?'

'Oh. It's Mr Reynolds who's got a really bad chest, who had a hernia repair under local this morning. He's had some paracetamol which hasn't helped and he's in severe pain every time he coughs.'

'Isn't he written up for anything stronger?'

'No, because they were afraid of sedating him too much, I think.'

Dr Peters muttered angrily under her breath. She hated getting out of bed for someone else's patient and resented losing any more of her precious sleep.

'Oh. All right. I'll come and sort something out.'

'Thank you doctor.'

Ten minutes later, an exhausted-looking Dr Peters shuffled onto the ward and asked for the case-notes. Sighing wearily, she followed the sounds of coughing and laboured breathing to find John in some distress.

'Doctor. . . thank you. . . it hurts. . . here. . .,' he gasped between wheezy breaths. She examined the wound to make sure it hadn't given way. John was too distressed to feel embarrassment.

'Are you usually this short of breath?' she said, pulling her stethoscope out of her pocket.

'No, doctor. . . It's bad tonight. . . and the pain!'

Dr Peters listened to his chest and could hear wheezes and rumbling noises.

'Staff! We'll have to sort this out. Can you get me his drug chart please. . . I see he's already having the nebuliser and antibiotics. How much relief do you get from the nebuliser, Mr Reynolds?'

'You mean. . . the mask treatment?. . . It's good. . . but it doesn't last long.'

'OK. Staff, I want to give a stat dose of nebulised salbutamol, 2.5mg, and I'll increase the frequency to four hourly. I'll write up a stat dose of pethidine and he can have it three hourly. That might help a bit with the wheezing as well.'

'Mr Reynolds, we'll give you a pain-killing injection which will probably make you rather sleepy and might depress your breathing a bit. So it's very important that you keep an oxygen mask on through the night. And we'll give you an extra dose with the nebuliser.'

'Thank you, doctor. . . Sorry. . . to disturb you.'

'That's OK.'

'Staff, I'll speak to Andrew in the morning. We need to sort something out to provide better pain relief so that Mr Reynolds can cough properly.

Oh, make sure that it's a 24% oxygen mask because we don't want to give too much.'

Later that morning, Andrew, the houseman, phoned Dr Lewis to ask for his help.

'Sorry to bother you. It's about Mr Reynolds who had his hernia repair done under local yesterday. I know you weren't involved in his care but we've got a real problem with pain relief and I wondered if you could do a nerve block or something. He's got very severe bronchitis and the pain is stopping him from coughing and clearing his chest. The physiotherapist saw him earlier and she's quite worried.'

'OK, Andrew, I might be able to make time at the end of my morning list. Sounds like we ought to try an ilio-inguinal block first and we can always think about an epidural later. I won't have much time so can you get me some things ready. I'll want a syringe, needles and 20ml of 0.5% bupivacaine. What ward is he on?'

He came a little before one o'clock. John lay on his bed while Dr Lewis felt for a prominence on his hip bone above the right groin. Moving a little towards the midline, he advanced the needle perpendicularly through the skin until he felt it penetrate a fibrous layer in the abdominal wall. He then injected the local anaesthetic just under this layer and withdrew the needle.

'The two main nerves that supply the groin region lie just under the external oblique aponeurosis,' he explained to Andrew. 'If we block those, we can relieve about ninety percent of the pain.'

'Mr Reynolds, it should start to go numb in the next few minutes and take most of the pain away. It'll last most of the rest of today and we need to take advantage of that to work on your chest and clear the sputum. Hopefully, by tomorrow, it won't be so bad.'

'Thank you doctor. . . It's starting to feel. . . better already.'

PAIN RELIEF AFTER OPERATIONS

This is a subject of great concern to almost everyone having an operation. As we have seen from the experiences of George and John, analgesia can sometimes be inadequate. Susan, on the other hand, has superb pain relief by the use of more sophisticated techniques. I would like to discuss this subject while the examples are still fresh in your mind. But before I go on to describe the different methods of pain relief in common use, it is worth considering some of the general features of pain and the principles of analgesia.

Pain is wholly subjective. It is an individual experience that cannot be measured by any external test or device. The experience of pain has several components. An injured part of the body transmits signals to the brain

Post-operative Recovery · 125

which are interpreted as pain. These signals travel by different nervous pathways, at different speeds of conduction and so arrive at different times. Thus if you were to drop a brick on your toe and concentrate carefully on the resulting sensation, you would notice that an initial sharp sensation was followed by a second wave of duller burning pain. Thus there are 'fast' and 'slow' components of pain, separated in time. Often the fast pain triggers a rapid reflex withdrawal of the injured part and this reflex action may begin before the brain has time to register pain. An example of this is the reflex withdrawal of your hand if you accidentally touch something burning hot. Pain may also induce a variety of other protective reflexes, such as muscle spasm, which attempt to protect the injured part. Thus acute appendicitis leads to spasm of the muscles of the abdominal wall and a slipped disc causes intense muscle spasm in the back.

Pain is also associated with an emotional response which can itself greatly modify the perception of the pain. For instance, fear and anxiety heighten the perception of pain whereas mental relaxation reduces the perceived pain. Some types of pain are associated with autonomic reflexes which can cause nausea, vomiting and sweating. This is particularly true of pain arising from the internal organs.

Pain is caused by a variety of insults but the two of greatest relevance to surgical patients are those of direct tissue damage and chemical inflammation. The two are never entirely separate as tissue damage almost inevitably leads to an inflammatory process triggered by the release of various chemical factors.

The net result of all this complexity is that the experience of pain can be modified in many different ways. Pain-killing drugs and techniques are targeted at different parts of the system and not all are effective for all types of pain. The following principles have been discovered:

1. Pain is increased by fear, anxiety and uncertainty.
2. If pain is completely relieved by a large enough first dose, then a re-occurrence of the pain can be prevented by regular smaller doses of pain-killer. The same smaller doses will be ineffective if the patient is already in pain. As a consequence, continuous pain relief can be achieved with smaller total doses of pain-killer than intermittent pain relief.
3. Pain is more bearable if you know it is going to end.
4. Side-effects of pain-killers such as nausea and constipation can be prevented if anticipated.
5. Powerful pain-killers such as heroin (diamorphine) and morphine are not addictive if used for the treatment of pain.
6. Pain originating from bone, muscle, joints or ligaments often responds well to anti-inflammatory types of pain-killers.

7. The route of administration of the pain-killer must be chosen to suit the circumstances. For instance, pain-killing tablets by mouth are no use in a patient who is vomiting.

8. Simple physical measures such as the splinting of a painful part may produce much relief of pain.

What happens in practice?

Sadly, much of the prescribing of pain-killers in our hospitals ignores these simple principles. This is not so much through ignorance as a lack of resources in the NHS. Let me illustrate this with an example.

The standard prescription for post-operative pain relief following medium or major surgery is papaveretum, by intramuscular injection, four hourly, as required. This drug is a natural mixture of compounds of which morphine is the main active ingredient. Morphine and the large series of related drugs are powerful pain-killers with a variety of important side-effects. They all cause varying degrees of sedation, drowsiness, nausea, constipation and depression of the breathing. The side effects are dose dependent and tend to disappear with repeated dosage. A drug to prevent sickness is also usually prescribed with the first few doses of papaveretum. A single injection into muscle has an effect within thirty minutes, a peak effect at about ninety minutes, and lasts three to four hours. Repeated doses have a more prolonged action but individual response is very variable. Morphine and related pain-killers are more effective against constant background ('slow') pain than sharp pain. Thus while a patient keeps still, good analgesia is achieved, but coughing or moving will cause sharp ('fast') pain in a wound which is less well suppressed by morphine.

In an ideal world, there would be enough nurses on the wards to ask every patient every four hours if they needed any more pain-killer. There would also be enough nurses to double check each prescription (according to the regulations) and administer the injections, also every four hours. This does not happen. In practice, most NHS wards are under staffed and the nurses are very busy. Pain-killers are often not administered unless a patient calls for attention and asks for them. There is then usually a delay before a second qualified nurse can be found to check the drug. Even when the injection is given, it takes up to half an hour to work.

Thus the phenomenon of 'break-through' pain occurs in which the last dose of pain-killer wears off before the next is given. It is theoretically possible for a doctor to circumvent this situation by prescribing a regular, timed dose of pain-killer. This would work for one or two patients but would be impossible to implement for a larger number.

The doctor who is primarily responsible for prescribing post-operative pain relief is your anaesthetist. Anaesthetists in general are expert at the theory and practice of pain relief and realise the shortcomings of the standard practice. Many will try and employ alternative measures.

One possibility is the use of a motorized syringe pump to deliver a constant stream of pain-killer into an intravenous needle. This system is very good at providing constant pain relief but has its problems. Firstly, the equipment has to be available. Secondly, the syringe contains a potential overdose of pain-killer, were it accidentally to be administered all at once rather than gradually over many hours. This means that a patient with such an infusion needs to be monitored closely and this requires close observation by nursing staff. This is not always possible on a busy, under staffed surgical ward.

An even more sophisticated system is a computerised dispenser which administers small doses whenever the patient pushes a button. This is programmed with a number of safeguards that prevent the patient getting an overdose. This system works very well and is liked by patients because they feel in control of their own pain. Unfortunately, the equipment is expensive and rarely available in the NHS.

Another approach used by anaesthetists is the use of longer acting local anaesthetic to block the pain from a surgical wound. An example of this is the nerve block that John had for his hernia repair, the day after operation. An extension of this is the use of a continuous epidural infusion such as Susan enjoyed. This technique can provide superb pain relief, without any drowsiness or sickness, but isn't widely available. Not all anaesthetists are familiar with the technique of inserting an 'epidural'. The surgeon will be kept waiting the ten or fifteen minutes it takes to set up an epidural before the operation and this time may not be available on a busy operating list. Formerly, this continuous epidural technique was reserved for patients closely monitored on an intensive care unit. There still persists a view, in many hospitals, that epidurals are complicated and hazardous and their use is prohibited on the general surgical ward.

The provision of post-operative pain relief is therefore a compromise. The more sophisticated techniques tend to be reserved for patients having major surgery or cases where effective pain relief is important to prevent complications such as chest infection. Most other patients get reasonable pain relief most of the time. Few operations produce much pain for very long and simple analgesics such as aspirin or paracetamol, taken regularly, are soon all that is needed.

Two particular sorts of pain-killer deserve a mention at this stage. There is a powerful pain-killer closely related to morphine called buprenorphine (brand name, Temgesic, a trade mark of Reckitt & Colman). This drug has been tailored so that any dose, above a certain threshold dose, will have the same effect, no matter how much is given. This makes the drug very safe, as a moderate overdose won't have any harmful effects. It also has an unusually long duration of action and a single dose will last six to eight hours. It comes in small tablets which are dissolved under the tongue, leading to a very rapid onset of action. Despite all these important advantages, the drug is not very commonly used. This is because the drug has a reputation of causing a high incidence of nausea and an unpleasant disturbance of the state of mind. This is certainly the case in some patients, particularly the elderly, but in others it produces very good analgesia without significant side effects and avoids the problem of break-through pain. I think it's worth a trial and if necessary, an anti-emetic can be given to prevent nausea. Temgesic is available on every surgical ward and this is something which you might like to discuss with your anaesthetist.

The other type of pain-killer I wanted to mention is that known generally as a NSAID. This stands for Non-steroidal Anti-inflammatory Drug. (Steroids have a very powerful anti-inflammatory action which is mimicked by NSAIDs, without any other steroidal action.) This is a broad class of drugs which are very widely prescribed for the pain of arthritis and other inflammatory conditions. The pain of some operations, particularly those involving tissues connected to the skeleton such as muscle and joint, may respond well to these drugs if they are started before the operation. These drugs do not produce any drowsiness, sedation, or depression of breathing, and their main side effect is a possible irritation of the stomach. The use of NSAIDs in post-operative pain relief is a growing area of research and is also a possibility which you may like to discuss with your anaesthetist.

Despite the short comings of post-operative pain relief in our hospitals, actually few people complain about this aspect of their stay. The pain of a surgical wound diminishes very rapidly if that part of your body is rested. Even after major surgery, very few patients ask for the powerful pain-killers for more than a couple of days.

DAY TWO

Unless you have had minor surgery, you are unlikely to notice many other symptoms on your first day. Like George, you will probably doze much of the time and you may not remember much of your first day. So we will now follow progress during the second day when pain is waning and symptoms such as 'wind' and a sore throat become more intrusive.

George

This was the day George began to feel human again. In the middle of the morning, two nurses came and gave him a bed bath. The whole of his skin was gently washed with a flannel and then dried and powdered. This was done in easy stages and to wash his back, they gently rolled him first onto one side then the other. George had been frightened to move in case the stitches broke but he was assured that every wound is closed with very strong stitches and he was quite safe to move or cough; there was no danger of the wound bursting open. When the bed bath was finished, George was surprised to discover that he was lying on clean sheets. The clean sheet was rolled half into position when he was on one side, and swopped for the soiled sheet when he was turned on the other side. He was able to clean his teeth and had a shave.

His tummy wasn't nearly so sore, and if he kept still, he could do without the pain-killers for longer periods. He was asked if he would like to sit out of bed in an armchair. At first, he was afraid of the pain of moving but when the nurses explained how they could lift him, he agreed. The effort was worth it and he felt much better sitting out. The chair was huge, soft and comfortable. The back reclined and a foot-rest came out of the bottom. George spent most of the day in the chair and it made it much easier to take the sips of water he was now allowed. Although he felt quite awake and alert most of the time he didn't have the energy to do anything and wasn't interested in reading. He watched the comings and goings on the ward.

During the day his belly began to feel rather bloated. He began to have a griping pain and could hear his tummy rumbling from time to time. Eventually, he broke wind several times and although this was embarrassing, at least the griping pain was relieved.

The physiotherapist came again and worked on his chest. The deep breathing and coughing was easier now and George felt no resentment. She was pleased with his progress.

Late in the afternoon, he was put back in bed and feeling weary, stiff and sore, asked for a pain-killing injection. He slept much of the evening and through the night.

Susan

Susan was given breakfast in bed and then her epidural tube was taken out. She was slightly nervous that this would hurt but the worst bit was peeling the sticky tape which ran right up her back, and over her shoulder. The tube came out easily with no more than a slight twinge. She was allowed to walk carefully to the bathroom for a bath and when she came back, her bed had been moved to a quieter bay away from most of the hustle and bustle of the ward. Susan wanted to know why she couldn't go home that day.

'Don't forget, you've had quite a big operation and we need to watch out for complications. We'll be keeping a careful eye on your temperature and we want to make sure you don't develop a leak of bile from where the gall bladder was removed. You need to rest and you won't get that if you're home with the children.'

Later in the day, Susan began to realise that her wishes for discharge were premature. It took some hours for the effects of the epidural to wear off and her wound became increasingly tender. When she moved, she felt a very sharp pulling sensation from one end of the wound and although she was comfortable most of the time, this restricted her mobility.

John
The worst was over now, with a combined improvement in his chest and a lessening of the pain in the wound. The physiotherapist had taught him how to protect the groin while coughing, by pulling his right thigh up towards his tummy. John was encouraged to get up and about and was discharged from hospital the next day. His recovery was otherwise very straightforward and he had been able to eat and drink almost immediately after his operation, a benefit of local anaesthesia. He didn't need any drips or tubes. Before he went, he was advised not to drive a car for several weeks.

'Your insurance will be invalid until the groin has healed and isn't painful any more. This is because the pain might stop you using the brakes properly in an emergency. Also, you mustn't do any lifting for two months so as not to strain the repair.'

OTHER COMMON POST-OPERATIVE SYMPTOMS

Sore throat
This is a very common complaint. Unless you are having a minor operation, it is quite likely that the anaesthetist will control your breathing during the operation by inserting a tube into your windpipe. This can cause a sore throat that may persist for some days.

Wind
Patients sometimes find this very uncomfortable and embarrassing. The problem occurs after abdominal operations and if powerful pain-killers are prescribed. As I explained in the sections on drips and tubes, if the bowel is handled or operated on, it tends to go on strike. Fluid and gas accumulate and can lead to painful distension. Pain-killers like morphine make the problem worse because they inhibit bowel action. Epidurals avoid this problem and the bowel recovers more quickly, allowing patients to eat again sooner after their operation.

A remedy popular on the wards is peppermint water which acts as an antispasmodic. Otherwise, the discomfort has to be borne until it sorts itself out naturally. Don't be too embarrassed if you get a lot of wind. This is very common on the ward and the staff will understand that it is a side effect of the operation.

Muscle pains and stiffness

Anyone confined to bed for several days will get stiff and sore. In addition, if you have had a long operation, the awkward position on the operating table may lead to tender spots. However, some patients may experience severe muscle pains and stiffness, like a bad 'flu. This is a common side effect of a particular anaesthetic drug called suxamethonium. This drug is used to provide extremely rapid and profound muscle relaxation followed by recovery within a few minutes. It is used in certain emergency cases and also where intubation of the windpipe is required for a very short operation such as tonsillectomy.

Anaesthetists are well aware of this side effect which occurs in only a proportion of cases, and which is unlikely in the older patient. They will try and avoid the use of this drug wherever possible. Several major drug companies are investing heavily in research to find an alternative to the drug because of this side effect.

DAY THREE

George

The doctors came round as usual, soon after eight.

'How are you feeling, Mr Saunders?' asked the registrar. 'We're very pleased with your progress.' The houseman listened to his chest and tummy.

'Chest is clear, plenty of bowel sounds,' he reported.

'Legs all right?' enquired the registrar as he kneaded George's calves. 'Not tender?' George shook his head.

By this time, George was drinking well and the catheter showed a plentiful urine output.

'Time to take out some of these tubes, Mr Saunders. The drip can come down so long as you're drinking well, and the nasogastric tube can come out.' George looked intensely relieved. The stuck-in-the-throat sensation of the tube still almost made him gag.

'Have you been out of bed yet?. . . Then the urinary catheter can come out as well. Andrew,' to the houseman, 'keep an eye on that, will you? Make sure that Mr Saunders has passed some urine by the end of the day, otherwise you'll have to catheterize him again.'

'What about these drains? Much coming out of the superficial one now?

No? Then it can come out. Sister, have you a pair of scissors?' With a deft snip, he cut the stitch securing the smaller drain and, before George had time to react, he pulled the drain out.

'There! Didn't hurt a bit, did it?' Expressions of alarm and relief crossed George's face in rapid succession.

'I want to leave in the big drain for five days, at least, in case we get a leak. Nice and clean now,' he said, inspecting the bottle on the end of the drain tube. They passed onto the next bed.

George spent all that day sitting out of bed and took an interest in reading again. He felt very hungry but wasn't allowed anything except clear fluids. He was given a urinary bottle which was kept under an upturned paper bag on the bedside locker. By mid-afternoon he was beginning to feel uncomfortable but couldn't manage to pass any urine while reclining in the chair. He was embarrassed to mention it but the ward sister had kept a crafty eye on the situation and broached the subject herself.

'Mr Saunders, are you having trouble passing water? Don't worry, we'll sort that out. What we need to do is stand you up with your bottom on the edge of the bed.' She helped him up.

'Right. Get your bottle and I'll leave you to it.' She pulled the curtains around the bed and George stood with the bottle between his legs. No use! But then he heard the sound of running water from the sink beside his bed and the tension went out of his bladder. Slowly at first, and then with a satisfying stream, George was able to empty his bladder.

'Thank you, sister.'

'Usually does the trick!' she said with a smile as she pulled back the curtains.

Susan

Susan fretted to be allowed home. She was eating perfectly normally and could now walk around the ward with little discomfort. Her wound was tender but didn't hurt at all if she kept still.

She decided to go for a walk across the hospital to the library. Returning to the ward with several books, she felt a tiredness quite out of proportion to the trivial exercise. 'Perhaps the operation has taken more out of me than I realised,' she thought.

DAY FOUR

George was able to go to the bathroom in the morning and have a proper shave and wash. He carried the drain bottle with him. Later in the morning he went into the ward day room and watched television for a while. He felt weak and shaky from the days spent in bed without food. He had lost weight and felt thin and empty. However, he noticed that his feet and ankles were beginning to swell and he became worried.

'Not to worry!' said the houseman. 'We see this quite often. The problem is you've been starved for so many days on top of the operation, the level of protein in your blood has fallen. That was confirmed by one of the blood tests I did yesterday. Normally, the protein draws fluid out of the tissues back into the blood stream. Because yours is a bit low, fluid is accumulating in the tissues. This is always worse in the lowest parts of the body. If you keep your feet up on a stool, it won't be so bad. It'll soon go away when we've fed you up a bit.'

DAY FIVE

This was George's big day. If all was going well, the join in his bowel should have healed enough to allow him to start eating again. When the doctors came round, the registrar explained that he wanted to do a rectal examination. George was asked to lie on his side with his pants down. He felt the cold jelly and then the gloved finger feeling very gently around inside his back passage.

'Good. The suture line feels intact. No fever?. . . Abdomen soft, no tenderness?. . . Right! I think we can start feeding you now. Sister, light diet please.' She changed the notice on the head of George's bed.

'Andrew, can you contact the dietician please and arrange a high protein diet?' The houseman made a note in his book.

'Sister, could you take the big drain out today?'

'Very pleased Mr Saunders. It's gone very well. I had the histology report back from the laboratory this morning and the resection lines are clear. Also it's well differentiated.' George thought this was probably good news but didn't really understand what the words meant. The houseman explained to him later.

'When we remove a piece of tissue, we always send it to the histology lab to examine under the microscope. They process it into very thin slices which they stain and examine under the microscope. The tumour cells are different from the normal bowel cells so they look to see how far it's spread. In your case, it's well clear of the cut ends of the bowel, so it looks as if we got it all out. Also, the type of tumour cells they found were not too far removed from normal bowel cells so that increases the chance of a cure as well.'

'But it was cancer, doctor?'

'Yes, it was cancer, but I think we've caught it early enough and you have a very good chance of a complete cure.'

'Oh, thank you for explaining it doctor, you've put my mind at rest.'

Not only was George allowed to start eating that day but he was also allowed a bath, a great luxury.

'What about the plaster, Sister? Does it matter if I get it wet?'

'No. Don't worry. It's waterproof and it doesn't matter if it starts to come off. The skin will be healed underneath.'

George closely examined his wound for the first time while he was in the bath. It was covered with a transparent dressing, rather like cling film, but self-adhesive. He could see the line of the cut which showed up black where some blood had dried. There were also several areas of brownish-yellow discoloration on either side of the wound. George was puzzled that he could see no stitches but at each end of the wound, small plastic beads were fixed on the end of a nylon thread which disappeared into the skin. He later learned that this was a continuous subcuticular stitch that zigzagged under the surface of the skin. The day before he went home, one of the beads was cut off, and the smooth nylon stitch pulled out of the other end with a gentle tug. It didn't hurt at all and George was surprised at the length, almost eight inches. When the dressing was peeled off, all the black discoloration of the skin washed off leaving the scar as a neat, thin, red line.

Susan

Susan was allowed home on the fifth day. The doctors ran through a brief check-list in the morning. No fever, eating all right, bowels open and no tenderness in the legs? Her wound was inspected and she was told to attend her family doctor on the tenth day to have the stitches removed.

'When can I go back to work?' she asked.

'We'll make an appointment for you in the clinic in six weeks and I think you should stay off work until then. You'll be surprised how tired you feel when you get home and it would be a mistake to rush back to work. Take things easy but get some regular gentle exercise.'

DAY SIX ONWARDS

George was in hospital ten days altogether. His progress was rapid once he was freed of all the tubes and allowed to eat. He regained strength gradually, and put back a few pounds of lost weight. He was given a gentle laxative to ensure his bowel motions would remain soft and he passed stool for the first time on the seventh day.

The day before he went home, Mary brought in his clothes and he was allowed to dress and take a gentle stroll around the hospital corridors. He felt a return of some dignity as he dressed for the first time since coming into the hospital. He allowed himself to believe, for the first time, that life would go on and a future beckoned. He held Mary's hand as they walked along, something they hadn't done for many years.

YOUR TREATMENT MAY DIFFER

This chapter has been largely descriptive. I have tried to give you some flavour of the early days of recovery after an operation and your own progress will follow the same broad outlines. Many details will differ. No two patients and no two surgeons are exactly alike. Each surgeon will have his own set of rules governing the use of drips and tubes, early or late mobilisation, and time of discharge from hospital. Patients with the same diagnosis may have differing operations depending on their exact condition. So you cannot take as gospel the management of the four patients in this book nor should you criticise your own post-operative treatment by comparison.

The next chapter gives you advice on making a rapid recovery, avoiding complications and getting an early discharge home.

10 Discharge and Convalescence

Every patient should aim for a speedy and uncomplicated recovery. Few people like staying in hospital. After a major operation, you can advance your date of discharge if you have a positive attitude to recovery and follow some simple advice.

The behaviour of patients after an operation lies on a spectrum between two opposite stereotypes. In the second chapter I called these 'loungers' and 'go-ers'.

Loungers stay in bed as long as possible, complain of constant pain, demand repeated doses of pain-killers, and fail to co-operate with physiotherapists. They get complications. Their prolonged immobility places them at risk of venous thrombosis and chest infection. The repeated doses of painkiller delay their recovery by inhibiting the bowel which remains on strike, resulting in nausea, loss of appetite and constipation. Because they can't eat or drink, they feel weak and unwell. The drip has to be continued longer. All these factors can delay wound healing. A vicious circle may develop, leading to serious illness and a prolonged stay in hospital.

Go-ers have a radically different attitude. They can't wait to be up-and-about and prefer to be alert and interested, if in some discomfort, rather than sedated with prolonged use of powerful pain-killers. They co-operate fully with the physiotherapists and do the breathing and limb exercises enthusiastically. Go-ers are constantly asking, 'When can I drink? When can I eat? When's the drip coming down? When can I go home?'

Of course, if you are elderly or have had a very serious illness, you may need a longer stay in hospital to recover and regain your strength. But this doesn't alter the great importance of your attitude to recovery and the quicker you make your early recovery, the sooner you can begin to build up strength again.

COMPLICATIONS

This is a word that has cropped up repeatedly. To remind you, a complication is an undesirable side effect of an operation, anaesthetic or treatment. Complications can be divided into two groups, those that are associated with the particular operation, and those like infection, bleeding or thrombosis that might occur after any operation.

Usually, the specific complications are related to the technical aspects of the surgery and arise out of natural difficulties or mishap. There is little the patient can do to influence this. General complications, on the other hand, do depend on the attitude and behaviour of the patient post-operatively. Two such complications are particularly important and you ought to know about these, although I have referred to them before. I will consider each in turn.

Deep venous thrombosis (DVT)

Thrombosis means formation of a blood clot. During an operation and anaesthetic, a number of things happen that make thrombosis more likely in the deep veins of the legs and pelvis. General anaesthetic agents disturb the delicate balance between formation and dissolution of blood clots, making clotting more likely. Flow in these veins stagnates due to immobility of the patient and compression of the veins during the operation. The disease process itself may change blood coagulability and also make clotting more likely. The net result is that up to 40% of patients develop some degree of deep vein thrombosis after abdominal operations. This is not usually clinically obvious and this figure comes from studies using sophisticated body-scanning techniques to detect small clots.

So why does this matter? Usually, it doesn't but there is a slim possibility that a blood clot may peel off the wall of a vein and travel up through the heart. When it reaches the lungs, the clot impacts in a blood vessel and prevents blood flow to that segment of the lung. A small clot causes chest pain and a slight reduction in oxygenation of the blood. A very large clot is instantly fatal, as it blocks the entire blood circulation. Intermediate sized clots may make a patient seriously ill with a severe reduction in the oxygen content of the blood and a serious strain on the heart which tries to pump past the blockage.

Certain groups of patients are particularly at risk, including for instance, the elderly and patients having hip surgery. The risk is also increased if you are taking the contraceptive pill. In numerical terms, the risk is very small but you may still be advised to stop the pill before a major operation, for this reason.

Surgeons and anaesthetists are very well aware of the potential dangers of DVT and, in the higher risk cases, will take a number of precautions. These include surgical compression stockings, thinning of the blood with injections or tablets, and most importantly, early mobilisation of the patient post-operatively.

This last measure cannot be stressed too highly. Prolonged immobility after an operation allows a DVT to increase in size with possibly serious or even fatal consequences. For this reason, it is essential that you get moving as soon as possible after your operation and particularly that you keep the feet and legs active. The deep veins and muscles of the legs act as a blood pump to maintain flow in the veins. Whenever the feet or legs are moved, the muscle tension squeezes the veins, propelling blood back towards the trunk. Blood cannot flow the other way because of one way valves in the veins. The physiotherapist will instruct you in the necessary foot and leg exercises which keep the veins empty and prevent stagnation and clot formation. Posture is also important to prevent pooling of blood and if you are sitting out in a chair, you must keep your legs elevated on a stool. While lying in bed, you must not cross your legs as this compresses the calves, impeding blood flow.

Most DVT goes undetected but you should watch out for the signs of a thrombus in the leg. The signs are swelling, pain and tenderness of one calf, accompanied by puffiness of the same ankle. You must tell a nurse or doctor if you notice this. Sometimes, a small blood clot will travel to the lung without a thrombosis being obvious in the leg. This causes a very sudden and characteristic pain in the chest. The pain is sharp and stabbing in nature, and is worse when you breath in. The pain is well localized to one spot and you will easily be able to point to where you feel the pain. These symptoms are not exclusive to a blood clot in the lung and there are other quite innocent and trivial causes of this sort of chest pain so don't jump to conclusions. Whatever the cause of the pain, you should quickly tell a nurse or doctor. If you do have a clot in the lung, you may also become short of breath or even cough a little blood.

If there is a strong suspicion of DVT or of clot in the lung (pulmonary embolus) then the doctor will immediately start you on a drug called heparin which reduces the clotting tendency of the blood. This is given by continuous intravenous injection using a syringe pump. Each patient will need a different dose to achieve the same result so blood tests will be done daily to measure the effect on clotting. If a DVT or pulmonary embolus is confirmed by an x-ray or scan, you will be started on warfarin tablets, which have the same effect as heparin, but on a much longer time scale. Once the warfarin effect has built up over several days, the heparin will be stopped. Warfarin is usually continued for some months after an operation.

What happens to the blood clot? This is dissolved by a natural repair mechanism and eventually, blood flow returns to normal. No permanent harm is done. Heparin and warfarin do not dissolve blood clots but prevent any further extension of the clotting process. It is the active clotting process which causes the pain of a DVT, by setting up an inflammatory reaction. Once this is treated with heparin, the pain disappears very quickly although the clot may take days or weeks to dissolve.

The moral of the story is, get going after your operation and don't be a lounger!

Chest infection

This is commonest after abdominal operations but is unlikely in the young, non-smoking patient. Smokers, the elderly and the obese are at risk.

Whenever we breath shallowly, small areas at the base of the lung remain closed and unventilated. During and after an anaesthetic, because of changes in lung volumes, this effect increases and closed areas can collapse by absorption of trapped air. The mechanisms for clearing secretions from the airways are also inhibited, leading to blockage of small airways and further areas of collapse.

In the fit patient, these changes are quickly reversed by deep breathing exercises. However, if breathing remains shallow, bacteria can multiply in collapsed areas leading to chest infection or even pneumonia. Any abdominal operation will make breathing uncomfortable, more especially if a cut is made in the upper half of the belly. The pain will also inhibit coughing. Pain-killers themselves depress breathing. Thus, immobility, shallow breathing, failure to cough and the prolonged prescription of powerful pain-killers are a recipe for chest infection. Prevention of a chest infection, like prevention of venous thrombosis, depends greatly on the enthusiasm with which you do the breathing and coughing exercises. The sessions with the physiotherapist may be uncomfortable but are very important. Smokers are SIX times more likely to get a chest infection after abdominal surgery than non-smokers! You must try hard to give up smoking before your operation and if you can't, work hard at preventive measures after the operation.

So why does a chest infection matter? The effects are several: Any infection will cause a fever. Not only will this make you feel unwell but important reserves of energy are consumed and body tissues will tend to break-down rather than heal. A serious chest infection will reduce the amount of oxygen in the blood and this also delays healing. The continuous coughing caused by a chest infection places a strain on an abdominal wound and, in serious cases, this may be permanently weakened, leading to a hernia. Your stay in hospital will be prolonged and the antibiotics used to treat the infection may produce unpleasant side-effects such as diarrhoea or thrush (fungal infection of the mouth or vagina). Chest infections are preventable. Don't let it happen to you!

Wound complications

Most wounds heal rapidly and cleanly. However, it is not uncommon for one part of a large wound to heal more slowly and to discharge some fluid. If this happens, a small part of the wound may gape slightly when the stitches come out. This is no cause for concern as the wound is stitched in several layers and usually it is just the skin that has come apart. The deeper layers will be firmly held together and it is extremely unusual for a wound to burst altogether and require re-stitching. Sometimes a small hole may persist for some weeks, discharging fluid from deeper in the tissues. This is called a sinus and is treated with a daily change of dressing until it dries and heals naturally.

Wound infections are a more serious matter as they lead to tissue breakdown, rather than repair, and seriously weaken the wound as well as making the patient feel unwell. Usually the infection has come from a source of germs in the patient's own body such as a boil. Another possible source is infection from another patient or from a member of staff, transferred on unwashed hands. This is now very uncommon and should be entirely preventable. Diabetics and the obese are more at risk of wound infection.

If you do get a wound infection, the area will become red, hot and tender. A deep infection may make the wound swell like a boil and will eventually discharge pus. Any wound infection will be treated with antibiotics, usually given intravenously. If you have a serious infection, you may need to be isolated from the main ward and nursed in a side room to prevent the spread of infection to other patients. Any of the staff attending you will put on a gown and gloves to examine you or change dressings. Afterwards they will be careful to wash their hands before visiting other patients. This is not to say that the germs are highly contagious or dangerous to any fit person, just that other post-operative patients may be at risk. The sort of germs that cause these wound infections are carried by many of us on our skin. Visitors such as family or friends, from outside the hospital, are not at any risk and will not need to take the same precautions.

Most wound infections clear up well with antibiotics but your stay in hospital is likely to be more prolonged. At worst, your wound may need cleaning and re-stitching at a second minor operation.

The other possible complication in a wound is a haematoma. This simply means a collection of blood. A surgeon will be very careful to coagulate or tie every bleeding vessel in a wound but sometimes one will go undetected or will start bleeding after a wound is closed. This causes swelling and pain in a wound without the signs of an infection. The bleeding will almost always stop itself. A small collection of blood is a nuisance which doesn't justify any further treatment. It will eventually be absorbed but may leave a slight lump in the wound. A larger collection of blood will need to be evacuated in a second smaller operation.

Very occasionally, a wound will continue to bleed leading to significant blood loss or compression of surrounding tissues. This can be dangerous and will be dealt with urgently in the operating theatre. If blood loss is significant, a transfusion will be arranged to replace losses.

Complications are the exception rather than the rule. If there are any common or important complications associated with your operation, the surgeon should warn you about these in advance unless they are very rare. You can, of course, decline any such discussion if you feel it would make you unduly anxious before your operation.

Assuming you make a rapid and uncomplicated recovery, one question will be uppermost in your mind:

WHEN CAN YOU GO HOME?

The length of your stay depends on a number of factors but for any particular operation, your surgeon will have a schedule for normal recovery and discharge. This will be modified to take account of your fitness before your operation, how much support you have at home, and how well your early recovery has progressed.

In general, you will be allowed home when the following conditions have been met:

- You are mobile.
- You can eat and drink adequately and your bowels are working.
- You are mostly free of pain.
- That the high-risk period of complications has passed.

Your daily progress will be assessed by a system of surveillance on the ward with regular observations by the nurses and doctors. For instance, your temperature will be measured regularly to detect fever. The houseman will listen to your chest and examine your legs to exclude chest infection and thrombosis. Your wound will be inspected daily. Blood tests and x-rays may be done.

Over recent years, hospital stays have tended to get shorter. Partly this is a result of economic pressures leading to bed shortage; patients need to be discharged earlier to make way for new admissions. But this is also a result of improvements in both operative and anaesthetic techniques leading to a more rapid recovery. Even after the same operation, the length of stay will vary considerably between individual cases and between different surgeons. Typical examples (stay in days) might be:

Hernia repair	1–2
Varicose veins operation	1–2
Hysterectomy (removal of womb)	5–10
Major bowel surgery	10–14

142 · Discharge and Convalescence

Removal of gall-bladder (uncomplicated)	5–7
Total hip replacement	10–14
Prostate operation (transurethral)	4–6
Haemorrhoidectomy (removal of piles)	2–3
Tonsillectomy	1–2

ARRANGEMENTS FOR DISCHARGE

As the time nears, your surgeon should be able to give you a firm date for discharge. This is the time to start planning.

Clothes and personal belongings, sent home on admission, should be brought in soon before discharge. Any money or valuables in the safe keeping of the hospital will be returned at your request but may not be available at weekends when the administrative staff are off duty.

Prescription

If you need any medicines or tablets, these will be prescribed for you. In some hospitals, the hospital pharmacy will supply the tablets for you. In others, you will have to take a prescription to a chemist outside the hospital. (This is an attempt by the hospital to reduce spending on their own pharmacy department.)

Communication with your own doctor

You will be given a letter from the hospital to pass on to your GP. This is important, as your doctor has no other way of knowing that you have been discharged. It is best to deliver this letter to the surgery the same day. The letter will contain brief details of your diagnosis and treatment and will have a copy of your discharge drug prescription. If the houseman is particularly concerned about any aspect of your recovery at home, he will telephone your GP.

Outpatient clinic follow-up

If you are to be followed up in the outpatient clinic, you will be given an appointment card before you leave. Any patient having a major operation will be seen at least once for a progress check, usually six to eight weeks after discharge. Attitudes to the follow up of more minor cases vary and some surgeons like to see almost all their patients while others rely on family doctors to refer back any problems. The follow-up clinic is the last opportunity you have for expert specialist advice but it is very easy to forget half the questions you meant to ask. The best solution is to write down your worries or queries and take the list with you. Don't be afraid of wasting the doctor's time, he would rather your mind was put to rest.

Support after discharge

Sometimes, nursing care can be arranged at home, for instance to change surgical dressings. This will be done by the district nurse and you will be told of the arrangements. An elderly person who lives alone may require much more support in the way of home help, meals-on-wheels and so on. Sometimes, adaptations can be made to your home to make life easier. You may be taken on a home visit by the occupational therapists to anticipate any problems in advance. Patients are never just thrown out of hospital to cope alone and much trouble is taken by a large team of hospital staff to make sure you will be safe.

If you do live on your own and have had a major operation, then a short spell in a convalescent home can be arranged to help you recover your strength.

You should notify the local DHSS when you are going home so that pensions or benefits can be restarted. If you have any worries or queries about benefits, the hospital social worker will be able to help you.

How do you get home?

Most people will be expected to make their own way home after an operation. Ambulance transport is in limited supply and will be reserved for the elderly or needy. If you travelled to hospital by ambulance then one will almost certainly be arranged for your return journey.

A few days before discharge, the nurse in charge will ask you about travel arrangements. Most people have family or friends who can help and the ward staff will tell you where is the best place to bring a car to pick you up. A wheelchair to the pick up point can easily be provided.

You may be fit enough to travel by public transport but I wouldn't recommend anything except the simplest journey because after a stay in hospital, you will need time to adjust to the real world again. The simplest solution is a taxi.

After day-case surgery, you will not be allowed home unless accompanied. The after effects of an anaesthetic last many hours and include poor concentration, inco-ordination and forgetfulness. Even crossing a road can be hazardous when in this impaired state.

If you have a low income or are receiving state benefits, you may be able to claim back the cost of your journey to and from hospital.

STITCHES AND THE WOUND

Stitches have changed in recent years with the introduction of synthetic materials. A common type dissolves itself and so doesn't need to be taken out. This is placed entirely under the skin surface so isn't even visible.

Another type of stitch zigzags under the skin surface but comes out of each end of the wound, held in place by a bead. This is a continuous stitch make of a very smooth material which can slide in the skin. When it is time to remove the stitch, one bead is snipped off and the stitch is gently and painlessly pulled through from the other end.

Sometimes, the skin is closed with metal clips or staples but these would always be removed before a patient goes home.

The traditional type of skin closure, with a large number of individual stitches, is mostly favoured by orthopaedic surgeons who operate on the limbs.

How long the stitches stay in depends on the operation but almost always this is between five and ten days. If you are still in hospital, one of the nurses will remove the stitches. Otherwise your own doctor or the district nurse will do this.

Removal of stitches is a simple and painless procedure. The stitch is cut with scissors or a specially designed sharp blade and then gently pulled out with tweezers. Often a little scab or crust will be left where a stitch has come out. The first good soak in a bath will remove most of these and leave the wound clean and more comfortable.

For the first few weeks, the scar will show as a fine red line. Gradually this will fade and after about six months the scar will be the same colour as the surrounding skin, or slightly paler. Vertical scars in the abdomen will always be visible. Horizontal scars in the neck or lower abdomen lie in the natural plane of cleavage of the skin and heal almost invisibly.

For some weeks or months after your operation, you will often feel a pricking or pulling sensation in the wound when you move. This is nothing to worry about but is an indication that the internal healing processes are still taking place. Avoid movements, such as lifting, that cause this discomfort and this will protect the wound from excessive strain.

CONVALESCENCE

Before you leave hospital, you should ask the surgeon's advice about convalescence and return to work. The answer may surprise you. For instance, after an uncomplicated cholecystectomy (removal of gall-bladder) I would advise six weeks off work as an absolute minimum, even in a young patient. For reasons that are poorly understood, an operation is often followed by a prolonged period of fatigue and general lack of energy. Even though you may feel perfectly well and free of any discomfort or pain, you will quickly discover that trying to cope with your busy lifestyle takes a considerable toll. This is somewhat akin to the feeling of fatigue that can persist for some weeks after a bout of 'flu. In the early stages, even trivial tasks may lead to exhaustion. Feelings of depression are also common.

The more rest you can get in the early stages of convalescence, the better. For the mother with small children, this can be very difficult if not impossible, unless formal arrangements are made for alternative care of the children. Even if her husband takes time off work to help, a mother will get little rest unless the husband is a dab hand at cooking, cleaning and child minding.

For some people, the time of convalescence after a major operation provides a new perspective on life, and is an opportunity to re-examine life's interests and values. You may decide that your life has become unbalanced and that far too much time and effort is being spent on one occupation with neglect of others that might be more rewarding. Do you really need to work so hard? Personal relationships you have taken for granted might assume a new importance. A serious illness and then time for reflection can sort out the important from the habitual or trivial.

You should be given specific advice by the surgeon about daily activities such as driving. If your health is affected in any way which changes your ability to drive, you must report this to the licensing authorities or else not drive until you are completely recovered.

Advice about sexual matters is often not given, probably through embarrassment, but after a major operation you may be fearful of restarting normal sexual relationships. Probably the best time to broach this subject is at the follow-up appointment in the outpatient clinic. As a general rule, by the time you feel like sex again, recovery will be well advanced and you will have nothing to worry about. If you have had an operation like hysterectomy, you may have many more specific worries about sexual matters but in this case the doctors will be prepared for queries on the subject.

A TRIBUTE TO THE STAFF

Before you go, make your farewells and give thanks to the staff who have contributed so much to the success of your operation and recovery. Working in the NHS is not easy, with staffing and resources stretched to the limit. The quality of care in our hospitals is a tribute to the dedication of the very large team involved in the care of each patient. Although a small gift, such as chocolates, is enjoyed, a greater reward is a card or letter expressing appreciation of the care you have received. It is also nice to know that the operation has been a success and that you are fully fit and enjoying life again. Of course, you may feel dissatisfied with some aspect of your treatment and the procedures for complaint are discussed in the final chapter. But do try to remember the other staff who have given you worthy service and make your thanks where they are deserved.

11 How to Complain and Sources of Help

The experience of going into hospital for an operation has many different aspects. Although most patients express general satisfaction with their treatment, you may have noticed particular deficiencies in the service or you may be unhappy with your medical treatment or operation. Often the complaint is about administrative matters, such as poor amenities or delay in treatment, which may be outside the jurisdiction of staff directly involved in patient care. Comments or complaints about different matters need to be directed to the appropriate person.

This chapter is a guide to your rights as a consumer in the NHS and how to go about making a complaint, either to obtain personal satisfaction or to improve the service for those who follow you. There are several agencies which represent consumer interests in the NHS and their role is described later in the chapter.

The hospital service is a complex organisation but responsibility for your care is mostly shared by three divisions: nursing, medical, and administrative. Day to day life on the hospital ward is overseen by the ward sister or senior nurse on duty. Worries or complaints about any aspect of your stay, with the exception of strictly medical matters, should be referred to the sister. Very often, a simple explanation will put your mind at rest and if there is some aspect of your nursing care that you feel is being neglected, prompt action can be taken to set this right. It is best to speak early rather than soldier on with increasing discomfort or resentment. You may have special needs that aren't apparent to the nursing staff and they will be glad to provide for these, once explained.

The so-called 'hotel' services of the hospital which include your accommodation, meals and amenities are the responsibility of the hospital administrators, as is much of the day to day running of the hospital. You may have been frustrated by the long wait in the outpatient department, a cancelled admission, poorly presented meals, restrictive visiting rules, inadequate bathroom facilities, or the lack of a telephone. Staff may have been rude to you, some personal item may have gone missing, or perhaps you suffered from a draught coming through a broken window. All of these matters can be referred to the hospital manager who has overall responsibility for the standard of service. The best approach is to discuss the matter with one of the ward staff first and they may be able to support your complaint.

You may also have suggestions for improvement of the facilities or service. Many hospitals provide cards for suggestions or comments and these are collected on the ward and sent to the hospital manager.

WHAT IF THE OPERATION HAS GONE WRONG?

The huge majority of operations are carried out exactly as planned without any mishap. Recovery is uneventful and the condition is effectively treated or cured. Occasionally, however, things do go wrong, for a whole variety of reasons. Usually this is not serious and the unexpected difficulties merely mean a longer operation than planned, or an extra stay in hospital. Let me give you some examples that occurred recently in my own hospital.

A middle-aged man had an operation involving his abdomen and urinary bladder. The operation was quite routine and straightforward. Because the surgery was expected to cause temporary bruising and swelling around the neck of the urinary bladder, some initial difficulty in passing urine might be expected. In accordance with routine practice, a suprapubic urinary catheter was inserted through the skin of the lower abdomen, to drain the urine. This catheter would be left in place several days and then removed. In addition, a soft rubber wound drain was inserted in the abdomen before the surgical wound was closed. Again, this was routine practice.

Two days later, the wound drain had done its job. The doctor on the ward cut the stitch securing the drain and gently pulled it to remove it from the abdomen. Usually, drain tubes come out very easily, with only a gently tug and without causing any pain. This drain would not come out, however hard the doctor pulled. Eventually, it was decided that the patient would require another operation to open the abdomen and free the drain tube. At operation, the answer to the puzzle was quickly discovered. By some incredible chance, when the suprapubic catheter was inserted through the skin, the introducing needle passed right through the soft rubber of the drain tube. The catheter transfixed the end of the drain, like a thread through a needle, anchoring it securely within the abdomen. Once the suprapubic catheter was removed, the drain came out easily.

This illustrates how things can go wrong by simple misfortune. The surgeon had taken all reasonable care and could not be blamed for this very rare occurrence. The patient required a second, minor operation but otherwise came to no harm.

Let me give you another example. This one illustrates how technical difficulties led to the dissatisfaction of another patient.

A woman in her thirties had completed her family and decided to be sterilised. This can be done in a variety of ways but by far the most common is laparoscopic sterilization in which the operation is done through a telescope inserted through a small cut in the edge of the belly button. This requires a brief anaesthetic but most patients have this operation as a day case.

During the operation, a needle is first inserted into the abdominal cavity and gas is blown in, under gentle pressure, to inflate the abdomen. This pushes the bowels safely out of the way allowing direct vision of the womb and fallopian tubes through the telescope. Each fallopian tube is identified and then sealed with a plastic clip which is clamped across the tube with a locking action.

In the great majority of cases, this is a simple and brief procedure. However, sometimes the fallopian tubes can be rather stuck down with old inflammation, or other organs in the abdomen can obscure the view. In this particular patient, one clip was easily placed but the second tube was difficult to reach. The second clip was locked onto the tube but the surgeon couldn't be 100% sure that the tube was effectively sealed. He then had a choice, and little time to make a decision.

The first option was to do a bigger operation, open the abdomen for a direct view and tie the second tube. This could be done under the same anaesthetic but the patient certainly couldn't go home the same day, the rest of the operating list would be delayed and the operation might be unnecessary anyway. The second option was to do no more at the time, but to arrange a special x-ray of the fallopian tubes at a later date to see if the second tube was sealed. The surgeon chose the second option and, later in the day, spoke to the patient and explained what had happened.

She was understandably disappointed at the possible failure of the operation and at the further inconvenience of having to attend for an x-ray. Disappointment later turned to dissatisfaction and anger, however. She was quite unprepared for the ordeal of the x-ray. This involved an internal examination, the discomfort and indignity of having a tube inserted through her cervix, and period type pains when the x-ray contrast fluid was injected through the tube into the womb and fallopian tubes. Unfortunately, to cap it all, the x-ray demonstrated that one tube wasn't sealed and she would need a second operation.

Being a professional lady of some means, she instructed her solicitor to sue the surgeon, alleging lack of reasonable care and failure to fully inform her of all the possible complications. She claimed damages for unnecessary suffering and for loss of income while attending hospital for the x-ray and second operation. When her solicitor sought an independent medical opinion, he was advised that there was no case to answer and that the surgeon had acted properly and in the patient's best interests, in these particular circumstances. The case was dropped.

I could go on with many more examples but this would probably only serve to frighten rather than educate. I have discussed the subject of complications in several chapters and I have also discussed the basis of the relationship between a doctor and patient, and what you can expect from your surgeon. Every surgeon recognises that operations can go wrong or have unfortunate side effects. These matters should have been discussed with you before your operation although some patients may choose to avoid the subject.

I would stress again that the huge majority of operations go perfectly well. The few that are complicated in some way are often the result of natural difficulties. Disease processes can take an unexpected twist or turn, and anatomy has unusual varients with unforseen results. The most remarkable example of this was a man who had two appendices. He developed acute appendicitis involving only one appendix. At operation, the first appendix was removed while the second appendix remained hidden. Some years later he presented again with severe abdominal pain and at emergency operation, an acutely inflamed appendix was found! The patient did not believe the story of two appendices, thinking instead that the first surgeon had negligently left behind his only appendix, instead of removing it. He tried unsuccessfully to sue.

A much smaller number of operations go wrong because the surgeon makes a simple and honest mistake, or an accident occurs during the operation. These problems are rarely serious and can almost always be put right. An even smaller number of operations go wrong because of negligence or lack of reasonable care by the surgeon. This is the only circumstance in which you have grounds to sue a surgeon and extract damages. These are the kind of cases that we read about in the newspapers from time to time. It must be realised that these cases are very rare, particularly when you consider that three million operations are done in the UK each year.

If you are dissatisfied with your medical treatment while in hospital, the best thing to do is discuss it with one of the doctors. The easiest person to approach is the houseman whom you will see on the ward every day. If there is a misunderstanding or your treatment was complicated by some natural difficulty or mishap, then the houseman will probably be able to satisfy you with a simple explanation. If you are still dissatisfied with your treatment and feel that you have received an inadequate level of care, then you must talk to the consultant who has responsibility for your care, or one of the other senior doctors on the firm. In these circumstances, the houseman is in a difficult position. He may believe that you have received poor treatment but is in no position to criticise his more senior colleagues. Without a good reference from his consultant, a houseman will be out of a job at the end of six months. Also, a houseman is relatively inexperienced and his opinion on the standard of treatment may not be expert. Any patient has the right to discuss his treatment fully and so if you feel strongly about the matter you should tell either the houseman or the ward sister that you wish to speak to one of the senior doctors.

This can usually be arranged quite easily although the doctor may not be able to see you the same day. Surgeons feel a very direct and personal responsibility for their patients and most will be anxious to discuss any problems with a patient. In the last few years, there has been a fast rising tide of medical litigation with ever increasing damages being awarded to victims of medical negligence. This has been reflected in a meteoric rise in the premiums all doctors have to pay for insurance against damages. This has focused doctors' attention on the need for good relations with their patients and the wisdom of full explanation if anything has gone wrong. So the majority of surgeons will attend promptly to any grievances.

Regional Medical Officer

If, after discussion with one of the senior doctors, you are still dissatisfied then there are various things you can do. The matter can be referred to the Regional Medical Officer, a senior officer of the Regional Health authority. This must take the form of a written complaint and must explain why you are still dissatisfied with the consultant's reply to your original complaint. The Regional Medical Officer will discuss the complaint with the consultant involved and will decide whether the full complaint procedure should be invoked.

This involves a complete review of the case by two independent consultants who will study all the case details. You will be interviewed and, if appropriate, a physical examination will be performed. Your interview and examination are private and completely confidential, and you are entitled to bring a friend or relative to support you at the interview. The independent consultants will also discuss the case with all the medical staff concerned.

A confidential report will be returned to the Regional Medical Officer, with recommendations for any action. Only the more serious complaints get this far but the procedure is not appropriate for those cases where legal action against the doctor or health authority is planned. The administrator for the health authority involved will then write to you and explain what action, if any, the health authority has taken as a result of your complaint.

Community Health Council

One criticism of the complaints procedure is that your complaint against the medical profession is being considered by other members of the same profession. Some patients feel that the procedure is therefore biased against them. There are, however, two completely independent agencies which represent consumer interests in the health service. The first of these is the Community Health Council (CHC). Each health district has a CHC which is independent of the local health authority. The members of the council include representatives of the local authority and voluntary organisations but not the medical profession. Although the CHCs have little direct power, they are widely involved in strategic health services planning and they are represented on various committees that actually decide where money is going to be spent. The CHCs solicit public opinion on major issues, such as closure of a hospital, and can mount publicity campaigns with considerable influence on health authority decision-making. They actively encourage dialogue between the health authority managers and the public they serve.

In England, the CHCs can also represent individual patients in complaints against the health service and will give valuable advice on the best way to proceed with a complaint about any aspect of the service. What they cannot do is make judgements about the clinical decisions doctors have made in your diagnosis or treatment. In disputes of this nature they can, however, help you present your case, steer you through the complaints procedure and give you advice on finding independent expert medical opinion, if this is appropriate.

They are eager to hear the views of any member of the public, be it praise or complaint, and they are always glad to hear suggestions for improvements in the service. The telephone number of your local CHC can be found in the phone book and often the address and 'phone number are given in the information booklet from your hospital.

Nationally, the individual CHCs are linked by the Association of Community Health Councils which has recently been campaigning for a charter of patients' rights. Their draft charter reads as follows:

All persons have the right to:
- health services appropriate to their needs, regardless of financial means, of where they live and without undue delay
- be treated with reasonable skill, care, and consideration
- written information about health services, including hospitals and community and general practitioner services

- register with a general practice with ease and be able to change without adverse consequences
- be informed about all aspects of their condition and proposed care (including the alternatives available), unless they express a wish to the contrary
- accept or refuse treatment (including diagnostic procedures) without affecting the standard of alternative care given
- a second opinion
- the support of a friend or relative at any time
- advocacy and interpreting services
- choose whether to participate in research trials and be free to withdraw at any time without affecting the standard of alternative care given
- be discharged from hospital only after adequate arrangements have been made for their continuing care
- privacy for all consultations
- be treated at all times with respect for their dignity, personal needs, and religious and philosophical beliefs
- confidentiality of all records relating to their care
- have access to their own health records
- make a complaint and have it investigated thoroughly, speedily, and impartially and be informed of the result
- an independent investigation into all serious medical or other mishaps while in NHS care, whether or not a complaint is made, and, where appropriate, adequate redress.

The ombudsman

Also known as the Health Service Commissioner, the ombudsman has the power to investigate any serious complaint about hospital services except those solely involving matters of clinical judgement. His office was established by an act of parliament to consider individual cases where a patient has suffered injustice or hardship because of failings in the health service. He will consider a wide range of grievances but only after you have brought the matter up with your own hospital and have given them reasonable time to investigate and reply to your complaint. Almost all of the patients' rights mentioned in the charter above fall within the ombudsman's jurisdiction. Your hospital administrator, CHC or Citizens' Advice Bureau can tell you how to refer a complaint to the ombudsman but this must be done within a year of the occurrence about which complaint is made. Unlike the CHCs which exist in every health district, the ombudsman has only a single office and is not involved in matters of health planning. The address is Church House, Great Smith Street, London SW1P 3BW.

OTHER SOURCES OF HELP AND SUPPORT

A great number of self-help organisations exist, both locally and nationally, which give support for patients with particular conditions or disabilities. For instance, you will find support groups for patients who have cancer, renal problems, a colostomy, mastectomy, heart surgery, laryngectomy or ileostomy, to name but a few. Your local Citizens' Advice Bureau will have details of local groups and if you are still in hospital, the staff will be able to put you in touch.

Glossary

Appendicectomy Removal of the appendix.

Arthroplasty Refashioning of a joint, usually by insertion of artificial joint components, as in total hip replacement.

Arthroscopy Direct visualization of a joint with a telescope inserted into the joint space. Commonly used to diagnose and treat cartilage injuries of the knee.

Biopsy Strictly, examination of tissue samples in the laboratory. Now usually meaning the operation to obtain such tissue samples. For instance, biopsy of breast lump.

Cataract A clouding of the internal lens of the eye, which progresses with age. Treated by surgical removal of the lens, often replaced with an artificial lens.

Cautery Coagulation of tissue or small blood vessels by the application of a red-hot wire. A treatment for recurrent nose-bleeds.

Cholecystectomy Removal of the gall-bladder, the operation for gallstones which form within it.

Colectomy Removal of all or part of the colon, the large bowel.

Colic Abdominal pain which originates in the bowel, typically occurring in regular waves, each rising to a crescendo of pain, then abating.

Colonoscopy Examination of the inside of the large bowel with a telescope inserted through the back passage.

Colostomy Creation of an artificial connection from the large bowel to the skin, diverting bowel contents into a collecting bag on the tummy.

Complication A second condition which may co-exist in association with a primary diagnosis, complicating the patient's illness. For instance, obstructive jaundice is a complication of gallstones. Also used to refer to the side effect of an operation or treatment.

Contraindication A symptom, sign or circumstance which indicates that a certain treatment would be unwise or hazardous. For instance, a boil on the leg contraindicates hip replacement because infection might spread to the hip.

Glossary · 155

Cyanosis A blue discoloration, most noticeable in the lips and tongue, indicating a lack of oxygen in the blood. Always a serious sign.

Cystitis Inflammation of the urinary bladder, usually caused by infection, which results in a constant desire to pass water. Cholecystitis is inflammation of the gall-bladder.

Cystoscopy Direct examination of the inside of the urinary bladder with a telescope inserted along the urethra. Performed under local or general anaesthesia.

Debridement Cleaning of a wound by cutting away dead or damaged tissue.

Diathermy Application of heat, generated by a high frequency electric current, to seal small blood vessels or cut through tissue.

Diverticulum A blind pouch or cul-de-sac spontaneously formed in the wall of a hollow organ, most commonly the bowel. Hence, diverticular disease.

-ectomy A suffix from the Greek ektome, cutting out. Hence colectomy, mastectomy, lumpectomy.

Ectopic Literally, out of place. For instance, ectopic pregnancy which occurs in the fallopian tube rather than the womb.

Elective An elective operation is that chosen and planned in advance, in distinction to immediate emergency surgery.

Endoscopy Examination of a hollow organ using a telescope which reaches the internal cavity. See under cystoscopy, gastroscopy, colonoscopy.

Enema Application of fluid via the back passage for the purposes of irrigation, diagnosis or medication.

Excision Literally, a cutting out. For instance, excision of a breast lump.

Fistula An unnatural connection between two hollow organs or between an organ and the skin. For instance, a gastrocolic fistula joins the stomach and the colon.

Gastrectomy Partial or complete removal of the stomach, the treatment for severe ulcers or cancer of the stomach.

Gastroscopy Examination of the lining of the stomach with a flexible telescope inserted through the mouth and down the gullet.

Gynaecology That branch of medicine concerned with conditions of the female reproductive system, but not including pregnancy and childbirth.

Haematoma A localized collection of blood.

Haemorrhage Literally, a gushing of blood.

Hemicolectomy Removal of the right or left half of the colon, the large bowel.

Hernia Rupture. An abnormal protrusion of part of an organ through an opening in a body cavity. In the commonest type, a loop of bowel slides down the inguinal canal in the groin.

Hyper- Prefix meaning above or excessive. For instance, hypertension means raised blood pressure.

Hypo- Prefix meaning under or deficient. For instance, hypoglycaemia means an abnormally low concentration of sugar in the blood, sometimes abbreviated to hypo'.

Hysterectomy Removal of the womb.

Ileostomy Creation of an artificial connection which drains the contents of the terminal small bowel (ileum) into a bag on the tummy.

Ileus Paralysis of the normal muscular propulsion in the bowel, leading to distension with gas and fluid. A temporary ileus is common after any abdominal surgery.

Indication Sign, symptom or condition which indicates the need for a particular treatment.

-itis Suffix meaning inflammation. For instance, appendicitis is inflammation of the appendix.

Jaundice Icterus. Yellow discoloration of the skin and eyes caused by an excess of bilirubin in the blood. Bilirubin, a waste product of red blood cell breakdown, is excreted by the liver. Jaundice may be caused either by excessive breakdown of red cells, or inadequate excretion due to disorders of the liver and gall-bladder.

Laparotomy Surgical opening of the abdominal cavity to perform an operation within.

Ligation To tie or bind with a thread. For example, tubal ligation is a method of sterilization where the fallopian tubes are tied.

Lipoma A soft, benign lump composed of encapsulated fatty tissue.

Lithotripsy Wearing away of a kidney stone or gallstone by repeated shock waves. This can now be done by a machine which focuses high intensity sound waves onto a stone without damaging surrounding tissues, thus destroying the stone and avoiding an open operation.

Glossary · 157

Lobectomy Removal of a lobe, for instance of the lung, or of the thyroid gland.

Lumpectomy Removal of a lump.

Mastectomy Removal of a breast.

NBM Nil by mouth. An abbreviation for the instructions given to patients before surgery.

Nephrectomy Removal of a kidney.

Oesophagectomy Removal of the gullet. A new connection to the stomach is made, either by moving the stomach into the chest, or by transplanting a segment of bowel to bridge the gap.

-oma A suffix meaning tumour. For example, lipoma, a benign tumour composed of fatty tissue.

Oophorectomy Removal of an ovary.

Ophthalmologist An eye specialist.

Orthopaedic Concerned with the locomotor system, the skeleton, joints and muscles.

-osis A suffix meaning a condition. For instance, asbestosis, a condition caused by exposure to asbestos.

Paediatrician A specialist in childhood illness.

-plasty A suffix meaning to refashion or form.

Pneumonectomy Removal of a lung.

Polyp A pear-shaped overgrowth of tissue, for instance of the bowel lining or nasal air passages.

Polypectomy Removal of a polyp.

Prolapse Abnormal protrusion of an organ into or through a natural orifice. For example, prolapse of the womb into the vagina.

Prostatectomy Partial or complete removal of the prostate gland which sits at the bladder neck. As the gland enlarges with advancing age, it can obstruct the outflow of urine. The treatment is prostatectomy, usually performed through a telescope inserted into the urethra. Hence TURP, trans-urethral resection of prostate.

Pyrexia Fever. A rise in body temperature above the normal thirty-seven degrees centigrade.

Resection Cutting out.

Sepsis Poisoning due to the products of infection. Septic shock (blood poisoning) occurs in severe sepsis when infection spreads to the blood stream.

Septoplasty Refashioning of the nasal septum, the midline structure of cartilage and bone which separates the two sides of the nose.

Stasis Stagnation. A loss of the normal flow or movement. For instance, venous stasis which may occur in varicose veins.

Suture A stitch.

Syndrome A collection of symptoms or signs which, when occurring together, form a recognised pattern indicative of a certain condition.

Thoracic Referring to the chest.

Thyroidectomy Removal of the thyroid gland from the front of the neck.

Tomography An x-ray technique that produces images of sections of the body, as if sliced like bread.

Tubal ligation A method of sterilization in which the fallopian tubes are tied.

TURP See prostatectomy.

Urethra The tube which leads from the bladder to the exterior, through which water is passed in the act of urination.

Varicose Swollen and tortuous.

Index

Abdominal weakness, exercises for, 28
Acupuncture, 91
Admission letter, 38
Admission
 to hospital, 40
 to the ward, 41
Alcohol consumption
 effect on anaesthetic, 34
 recommended limits, 34
 withdrawal, 34
 and vitamin deficiency, 34
Ambulance transport, 40
Anaesthetic, 78–92
 awareness during, 83
 epidural, 87, 107
 general, 78
 local, 84–89, 109–111
 pre-med, 49, 109
 pre-op visit, 49
 room, 105
 safety of, 81
 side-effects, 130, 131
 spinal, 88
Anaesthetist, 56
Anaemia, definition of, 67
Analgesia, definition of, 78
Ankle swelling post-op, 133
Antagonist, 90
Anticoagulants, stopping before surgery, 34
Antidepressants, interaction with anaesthetic, 35
Awareness under anaesthesia, 83

Barium enema, 70
Bed-bath, 128
Benefits, and admission to hospital, 39, 64, 143
Blood tests, 67–69
 avoiding a bruise, 67
 blood chemistry, 68
 blood count, 67
 kidney tests, 68
 liver tests, 68
Bowel preparation, 108
Bronchitis, risk of anaesthetic, 17, 33
Buprenorphine, 127

CEPOD, 82
CT scanner, 72
Caesarean section, awareness during anaesthetic, 83
Catheters, urinary, 116, 117
Chest condition, pre-existing, 27
Chest infection, 139
 and smoking, 33
 post-op effects, 139
 prevention, 139
Chest physiotherapy, 120
Cirrhosis, 34
Clerking, by the nurse, 42
 by the houseman, 43
Cold, the common, and postponing surgery, 28
Community Health Council, 151
Complaints procedures, 146–152
Complications of surgery, 136–141
 avoiding, 136
 chest, 139
 wound, 139
 pulmonary embolism, 138
 venous thrombosis, 137–138
Consent to operation, 93–103
 abortion, 101
 informed, 94, 95
 in practice, 96
 minors, 101
 refusal to accept transfusion, 101
 research, 102
 sterilization, 100
Constipation, 30
Contraceptive pill, stopping before surgery, 35
Convalescence, 143, 144
Cross-match, 68

Day case surgery, 49
Dental treatment, 35
 protection of crowns, 35
Diagnosis, principles of, 9–11
Diathermy, 106
Diet
 influence on healing, 29
 to lose weight, 31
Dietician, 63
Discharge from hospital, 141–143
 ambulance transport, 143
 conditions for, 141
 journey home, 143
 letter to GP, 142
 outpatient follow-up, 142
 prescription, 142
District nurse, 143
Doctors, 51–58
 anaesthetist, 56
 consultant, 54
 houseman, 52
 oncologist, 57
 physician, 57
 radiologist, 57
 registrar, 54
 senior house officer (SHO), 53
 senior registrar (SR), 54
Domestic staff, 64
Drains, surgical, 115
Drip, 106, 112

ECG (electrocardiogram), 76
Endorphins, 90
Endoscopy, 75
Enrolled nurse, 59
Epidural anaesthetic, 87, 107
Exercises in preparation for surgery, 28

Gamma camera, 74

Haemoglobin, 32, 67
Health Service Commissioner (Ombudsman), 152
Heart condition, pre-existing, 27
Heparin, 138
Hernia
 inguinal, 15–16
 incisional, 28
Histology, 133
Hospital manager, 147
Hospital staff, 51–65

IVP, 71
Identity bracelet, 42

160 · Index

Ileus, post-operative, 114
Inguinal canal, 16
Insulin, 34
Internal examination, 44

Jehovah's witness and transfusion, 101

Kidney tests, 68, 71

Length of stay, 141
Letter to GP, 142
Liver tests, 68
Local anaesthetic techniques, 84–89
  epidural, 87
  infiltration, 85
  intravenous regional, 86
  nerve blocks, 85
  plexus blocks, 86
  spinal, 88

MAOI, stopping before surgery, 35
MRI (magnetic resonance imaging), 73
Meals on the ward, 46
Meals-on-wheels, 64
Medications, consulting your GP, 35
Mental attitude, 25
  effect on pain, 92, 125
  importance for recovery, 26
Menu cards, 47
Minerals, importance for healing, 29
Mishaps during surgery, 147, 148
Mobilisation, early, importance post-op, 137
Mono-amine oxidase inhibitors, 35
Morphine, 89
Muscle pains, 131
Muscle paralysis during the anaesthetic, 79

NSAID, 128
Naloxone, 90
Nasogastric tube, 107, 114
Nicotine, effects on heart, 32
Nurses, 58–60
  auxiliary, 59
  enrolled, 59
  sister, 59
  staff, 58
  student, 59
  theatre, 60
Nutrition, importance in healing, 29

ODA (operating department assistant), 60
Obesity and risks of surgery, 30, 31
Occupational therapist, 62
Ombudsman, 152
Oncologist, 57
Operation
  anaesthetic room, 105
  journey to theatre, 105
  pre-op check-list, 104
  that goes wrong, 147
  under local anaesthetic, 109–111
Outpatient clinic
  follow-up after surgery, 142
  initial consultation, 11–12, 20–21

Pain
  components of, 124
  power of suggestion, 92
Pain-killers
  alternative types, 127
Pain relief, 124–128
  break-through pain, 126
  local anaesthetic, 127
  placebo effect, 92
  practice on ward, 126
  principles of, 124–126
Patient's rights, a charter, 151
Pension while in hospital, 39
Pharmacist, 63
Physical examination, 43
Physical fitness, 27
  preparation for surgery, 28
Physician, 57
Physiotherapist, 61, 119
Placebo response, 92
Porters, 65
Post-op symptoms
  muscle pains, 131
  sore throat, 130
  wind, 130
Postponing surgery, 24, 28
Pre-med, 49, 109
Prescription on discharge, 142
Pulmonary embolus, 35

Radiographer, 62
Radiologist, 57
Receptors, 89
Recovery ward, 106
Rectal examination, 44
Regional Medical Officer, 150
Retention of urine, 116

Safety of anaesthetic, 81
Scanners, 72–74

Sex after surgery, 145
Shivering post-op, 109
Sickle cell anaemia, 67
Sleeping pill, pre-op, 48
Smoking, risks for surgery, 32
Social worker, 64
Sore throat, 130
Spinal anaesthetic, 88
Staff nurse, 58
Steroids, 34
Stitches, 143
Student doctors, 48
Student nurses, 59
Suggestion, power of, 92
Suprapubic catheter, 117
Surgical firm, 52

Temgesic, 127
Tests, 66–77
  IVP, 71
  barium enema, 70
  blood tests, 67
  electrocardiogram, 76
  endoscopy, 75
  scanners, 72–74
  urine tests, 69
  x-rays, 69–71
Thrombophlebitis, 15
Thrombosis, post-op, 137
Transfusion, 68
Transport to hospital, 40
Tubes, 112–117
  drains, 115
  drips, 112
  nasogastric, 114
  urinary catheter, 116

Ultrasound scanner, 72
Urinary retention, 116
Urine tests, 69

Veins
  of legs, 15
  varicose, 13–15
Vitamins and healing, 29

Waiting list, 36
Ward rounds, 47
Ward routine, 46
Warfarin, 138
Wind, post-op, 114, 130
Wound complications, 139
  haematoma, 140
  infection, 140
  sinus, 140
Wound dressing, 134

X-rays, 69–71

WITHDRAWN